Prostate Cancer

Understanding the Causes and Treatment Options

(How to Defeat Prostate Cancer and Live a Long and Happy Life)

Brock Murphy

Published By **Tyson Maxwell**

Brock Murphy

All Rights Reserved

Prostate Cancer: Understanding the Causes and Treatment Options (How to Defeat Prostate Cancer and Live a Long and Happy Life)

ISBN   978-0-9959962-2-9

Legal & Disclaimer

The information contained in this book is not designed to replace or take the place of any form of medicine or professional medical advice. The information in this book has been provided for educational & entertainment purposes only.

The information contained in this book has been compiled from sources deemed reliable, and it is accurate to the best of the Author's knowledge; however, the Author cannot guarantee its accuracy and validity and cannot be held liable for any errors or omissions. Changes are periodically made to this book. You must consult your doctor or get professional medical advice before using any of the suggested remedies, techniques, or information in this book.

Upon using the information contained in this book, you agree to hold harmless the Author from and against any damages, costs, and expenses, including any legal fees potentially resulting from the application of any of the information provided by this guide. This disclaimer applies to any damages or injury caused by the use and application, whether directly or indirectly, of any advice or information presented, whether for breach of contract, tort, negligence, personal injury, criminal intent, or under any other cause of action.

You agree to accept all risks of using the information presented inside this book. You need to consult a professional medical practitioner in order to ensure you are both able and healthy enough to participate in this program.

Table Of Contents

Chapter 1: Prostate Cancer Can Also Be Called Carcinoma

The prostate This can be defined as the growth of prostate cancer Prostates are glands found in the reproductive tract of a male Chapter 2 of this book takes a thorough examination of the prostate as well as prostate cancer can bring majority of prostate cancers which occur inhibit the growth of other prostate cancers, but some tend to grow.

The cancerous cells are spread through the prostate region of the body, particularly the lymph nodes as well as the boneset first, it may cause no symptoms But, in the future, this issue can cause complications that are more complex, such as urine that is bloody and difficulty in urinating or discomfort in the pelvis or back.

Benign prostatic hyperplasia can be described as an illness that can manifest with similar symptoms to prostate cancer the other symptoms of late may be able to include tiredness because of the reduced levels of red blood cell.

However there is the possibility of cancer being a set of illnesses that cause cells that are abnormally growing and possibly spread to other parts of the body It is a frequent mistake to assume that all cancerous tumors are and this may not be correct Like cancer not spread, benign tumors do not across other body organs.

Some of the possible signs of cancer are irregular bleeding, inexplicably weight loss, lumps long cough, an increase in the frequency of bowel movements But, these symptoms could suggest an indication of the existence of cancer however there may be other causes behind the symptoms.

In the reports, up to 100 kinds of cancer may cause harm to an individual Around 22% of cancer-related deaths result from smoking cigarettes, while 10% of the statistics result from overweight, insufficient exercising, poor eating habits and consumption of alcohol.

Other causes of cancer are exposure to ionizing radiations as well as certain diseases and other environmental contaminants In the developed world 20% of all cancers are linked to illnesses like Hepatitis C and the hepatitis B as well as HPV (HPV).

The result is a change in the genes of a cell there are many mutations before it develops cancer However, can it also be passed down through the generations? Absolutely! Recent research has shown the 5-10 percentage of people's cancers are caused by genetic mutations inherited in their parents Cancer is diagnosed via specific signs or by a screening test.

Then, the issue is further investigated through medical imaging, and then confirmed through biopsyA biopsy is a diagnostic procedure performed by an interventional cardiologist surgical surgeon, or interventional radiologist, which involves the extraction of cells or tissues in order to assess the presence of cancer, or the degree of disease within the body.

Brief History of Cancer

Cancer's existence is just as old as the human race itself Documents available about the first discovery of cancer go as far back as 1600 Bit is believed that the Egyptian Edwin Smith Papyrus and the descriptions of breast cancer were the first documents to be documented.

Hippocrates identified various types of cancer in the period the 370 BC to in 460 BC and the Greek term for this was karkinos karkinos that means crab or crayfishThe term was derived from the cut-off surface of a malignant solid tumor that had veins expanding on each aspect, just like the crab's feet.

Regarding the perspective of cancer, a variety of theories have been developed over the course of time in an attempt to provide the most plausible genesis for the cancer tale Since the beginning of time doctors have been puzzled by the root causes of cancer It is believed that the Ancient Egyptians have blamed cancer on the gods We will look at a few of these prostate cancer theories.

The Humeral Theory

Hippocrates believed that the body was composed of four humor senses (bodily fluids) which included blood, phlegm (blood), the yellow bile and black Belief the humors are in balance and healthy, the person is in good health In this view that too much or small humor is the cause of illness The presence of black bile found in various organs was believed to trigger cancer The renowned physician Galen believed in this theory of cancer and was the Romans accepted.

It was the most accepted medical doctrine over a period of more than 1300 years in the Middle Ages Research in medical science was slowed due to autopsies as well as other studies of the body were banned on moral and religious grounds.

The Lymph theory

One theory which replaced the concept of humeral cancer was the notion that lymph, which is a different bodily fluid, triggers the development of cancer The bodily fluids of the body were believed to flow through our significant organs and tissues continuously, in order in order to create the life force The two major liquids are blood and lymph.

As per Stahl and Hoffman the cancerous cells are made from deteriorating and fermenting lymph which differs in acidity, density, and alkalinity The concept of lymph became popular John Hunter, a Scottish surgeon in the 17th century believed that cancers develop because of the lymph that is constantly released by blood.

The theory of Blastema Blastema theory

The year was 1838German Pathologist Johannes Muller proved that cancer was made out of cells, not lymphHe thought that cancerous cells did not originate in normal cellsMuller claimed that cancerous cells are derived from blastema which is a type of sprouting component, that's located between healthy tissuesHis pupil, the famous German pathologist Rudolph Virchow (1821-1902), found that all cells, including cancerous ones were derived from other cells.

The Chronic Irritation Theory

Virchow suggested that chronic irritation caused cancer However; he believed in the idea that cancer "spreads like a liquid." The work of a German surgeon by the name of Karl Thiersch demonstrated in the early 1860s that cancers are spread through the growth of malignant cells not by some mysterious liquid.

Trauma theory Trauma theory

Despite advances in the understanding of cancer, certain people believed that injury was the principal source of cancer in the latter part of 1800 through the 1920sEven though injuries were not likely to cause cancer in animals tested however, the belief accepted.

The theory of the Infectious Theory of Disease

Two Dutch doctors, Nicholas Tulp (1593-1644) and Zacutus Lusitani (1575-1642) both came to an identical conclusion about the spread of cancer almost in tandem.

Based on their own experiences of breast cancer within the same family They came to the Lusitania and Tulip created the theory of contagion popular in 1649 and 1652 as well Patients suffering from Cancer were kept in a separate area to stop spreading the disease, preferring to stay out of towns and cities.

History of Prostate Cancer

Niccole Massa, a Venetian anatomist was the first to define the prostate, in 1536An anatomist from another country, Andreas Vesalius, illustrated the prostate in 1538In 1853, the cancer of the prostate was recognized as a cancer of the prostate It was initially thought of as to be a rare condition, however the reason for this was poor screening techniques and lower life expectancy throughout the 19th century.

The first type of surgery was a method of treating prostate cancer It meant to eliminate urinary obstruction In 1904, the very first completely removing of the gland was done This procedure is called a radical prostatectomy It was done at Johns Hopkins Hospital by Hugh Hyosung.

However, the removal of tests (orchiectomy) via the operation for prostate cancer treatment was initially performed in the 1890sHowever, the procedure wasn't entirely successful Therefore that transurethral resections from the prostate area was suggested as a change to the process for radical prostatectomy.

One of the factors for this procedure was because it had better chances of keeping the penile erectile system Patrick Walsh was the person who invented the radical retro pubic prostatectomy procedure in the year

1983This procedure surgically was carried out to eliminate lymph nodes Charles Huggins, in 1941, published the findings of his study where he utilized estrogen to reduce testosterone production in patients with metastatic prostate cancer.

Charles Huggins won the Nobel Prize in Physiology or Medicine in the year 1966, for his breakthrough in chemical castrationRoger Guillemin and Andrzej WSchally determined the function of gonadotropin-releasing hormone (GnRH) in reductionThey were both awarded the Nobel Prize in Physiology or Medicine in recognition of their research on GnRH.

Chapter 2: The Prostate

The majority of men aren't certain exactly what their prostate gland is about The prostate is a tiny gland, and is a an integral part of male reproductive system It's size is similar to the shape like one of the walnuts The prostate is located just beneath the bladder and just in the rectum in front It covers a portion of the urethra tube inside your penis which is responsible for transferring urine out of the bladder.

The prostate assists in the movement of certain fluids within the semen It helps in transporting testicles sperm every time you exercise When you get older, your prostate grows larger This is typical for older menthe prostate's size can change from the size of a walnut into an apricot after an individual reaches 40 years in age By the time he reaches 60, the size of his prostate could be similar to an orange An enlarged prostate could squeeze the tube that is located in the urinary tract.

The problem can become very serious whenever one attempts to urinate It is normal for this to not be apparent until you reach the fifty-year mark or even older When one reaches the age of 50, there are three issues that can cause these modifications, and they include:

Inflammation (Prostitutes)

Benign Prostatic Hyperplasia (BPH) or an enlarged prostate

Prostate Cancer

Changes that take place in one person don't necessarily cause the other If, for instance, one suffers from prostitutes or benign prostate hyperplasia, this doesn't raise your chance of getting prostate cancer It is possible for people having several conditions simultaneously.

Many prostate problems that arise don't indicate cancer, contrary to what the majority of those who don't know are inclined to thinkThe following article will provide information on these conditions and the possible signs to help you understand these issues more clearly Let's get started! !

Inflammation (Prostatitis)

Prostatitis can be described as an inflammation or growth that occurs in the prostate glandIt can be caused by an infection caused by bacterialt affects about 50% of men at one time or anotherAs per the popular view that this condition can increase the chance of developing different prostate cancersHowever, this is a rumorThis condition doesn't raise the risk.

Types of Inflammation (Prostatitis)

Acute Bacterial Prostatitis

The main cause of this condition is bacterialt can happen abruptlyIn the range of types of inflammation, it's the most uncommon form of prostatitis, but it has serious signsThe patients suffering from this disorder are suffering from severe urinary tract infection that is coupled with an increase in urgency and frequencyUrination during the night can occur at night, and there's a sense of urgent need to urinate during those hours.

In addition it is also a source of pain that affects the pelvic and genital regionsIt is characterized by chills, fever nausea, vomiting as well as burning sensation when you urinateIt is important to treat this condition as it can cause prostate abscesses, bladder infections and obstruction in the flow of urineIf it is not treated the condition could result in lower blood pressure and confusion, and could prove deadlyIt is usually treated in a hospital setting with fluids, antibiotics and intravenous medications and pain relief medications.

Prostatitis chronically bacterial

The type of prostatitis described above is caused by a persistent infections in the urinary tract that allows access to the prostate glandIt is believed to be present for those who had this condition for many years prior to when it first began to show signsThe signs are similar to those previously mentioned (acute prostatitis bacterial).

There is only one difference: this kind of prostatitis isn't as serious and it can increase or decrease in severity with the course of timeWhen it is diagnosed, the condition can be challenging because it can be difficult for medical professionals to identify the bacteria present in urine.

The treatment includes antibiotics that can last from four to 12 weeksThere are instances where patients who suffer from this disease are provided with a suppressive, low-dose, and prolonged anti-biotic therapyIt's crucial to know that unlike acute prostatitis bacterial, it isn't a sudden occurrence and can become painful once it begins.

Prostatitis non-infectious and chronic

Of the three forms of prostatitisThis is the most common kind of prostatitis and it, according to research the disease accounts for a majority of all instancesIt is characterised by pain in the genital area and also urinary tract lasting for at least up to 6 monthsThe condition is common in males regardless of ageIt can be seen at the end of teens until old.

The symptoms can appear and go with no previous warningThe most common signs include discomfort in the groin or bladder region or discomfortTreatment for this condition can differ and is determined by signs.

The treatment may include pain-control treatment, anti-inflammatory medication and other medications like beta-blockers (used for relaxing the muscles' tissues that are located inside the prostate to facilitate the flow through the urine).

Prostatitis with symptoms of Inflammatory Prostatitis

It doesn't show any signs to it, therefore the majority of times, you don't consider it a kind of prostatitisThe condition is discovered in the course of an examination to determine different conditionsThe reasons that might require finding out include looking for prostate cancer and figuring out what causes infertilityFind out whether you suffer from this kind of prostatitis if you opt to the doctor for your prostate-specific test.

Benign Prostatic Hyperplasia (BPH) or an enlarged prostate

The term "Benign" means not cancer as such, whereas hyperplasia has something to do with an abnormal growth of cellsWhat happens is it is that BPH is a type of prostate that gets largerThe prostate condition isn't related to cancerIt doesn't add the likelihood of getting prostate cancerBut BPH has the same symptoms as prostate cancer.

BPH is among the leading causes of urinary tract problems and can be divided into voiding, storage and signsIt is a sign of urinary insufficiency.

The signs begin to manifest after 50It could include frequent urine flow and a slow or weak flow of urine, as well as the strain or pushing when the person begins to pass urineA larger prostate may cause pressure on the urethra and bladderThis can will slow or block the urinary flow.

After the flow of urine is started the process can be difficult to stop because some people are unable to complete the flow of urineSome experience a sense of urgency during the process of passing urineThis diagram illustrates what is explained in the previous paragraphs.

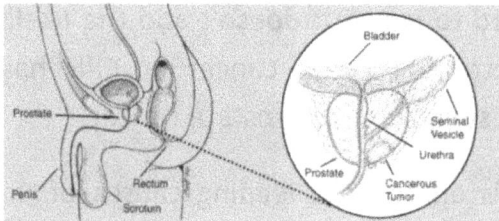

How to Treat BPH

People with BPH suffer from symptoms that can be a nuisanceIt is the worst thing about it that the condition is incurable however, the symptoms are reduced through surgical intervention or use of medicationsThere are three methods to control BPH.

Be on the lookout for

Therapy with drugs

Surgery

Watchful Waiting

Patients with mild BPH issues may not appear to have a lot of trouble, but the treatment may be necessaryBe patient and keep having annual check-upsThis checkup is termed"digital rectal examination "digital rectal examination," along with other tests that might be requiredTreatment is only initiated when symptoms get difficult to bearIf you're looking to undergo the wait and watch treatment follow a set of guidelines to follow that can assist in the reduction of symptoms.

There ought to be a restriction on drinking at night, particularly during the late at nightAlcohol or alcohol should not be consumed in the evening.

It should be a regular bathroom useIt means that you do not have to wait around for the bladder to empty.

Therapy with drugs

The majority of people suffering from mild to moderate BPH symptoms are choosing to use prescription medications instead of having surgeryTwo main types of medications can be used to treat BPH via the process of drug therapyOne drug performs its function by shrinking the prostate gland, while the second reduces the muscle tension around the prostateA few studies have been done and documented proving the consumption of both medications prevents symptoms of BPH from becoming worseThere are a variety of options to choose from.

Alpha Blockers

This type of therapy works by relaxing the muscles of the bladder neck and the muscles inside the prostateThis makes the process of urinating easierAlpha-blockers are doxazosin (Cardura) as well as alfuzosin (Uroxatral), Silodosin (Rapaflo) and Tamsulosin (Flomax)There are some side effects that can result from taking these medicines like dizziness, fatigue, and headacheA different side effect that can be encountered is an unintentional scenario wherein the semen flows back into the bladder, rather instead of ejecting from its penis point (retrograde Ejaculation).

5-alpha reeducates inhibitors

They aid in the reduction of prostate size because they stop the hormonal changes which cause the development of prostateThey help relieve symptoms by blocking the functions of an enzyme known as 5-alpha reductaseThis enzyme converts the hormone produced by male to dihydrotestosterone.

These drugs are dutasteride (Avodart) as well as finasteride (Proscar)Initially, the effects of the drug may not be evident due to the fact that it can take up to six months before they become active throughout the bodyThe adverse effect specific to this particular drug is is known as retrograde EjaculationAnother effect of this drug is less desire to have sexual contact and difficulty getting an sexual erection.

It is important to know that taking the drugs may reduce or reduce your prostate-specific antibody test results (we discuss this in the future)Research has concluded that consumption of these medications can reduce the chance of developing prostate cancerHowever, it does not stop the possibility of suffering from prostate cancerThe reason for this remains unclear.

Tadalafil (Cialis)

Research has suggested that the medication, employed to treat the condition of erectile dysfunction can assist in treating prostate growthHowever, it's not prescribed frequently and is only prescribed to men suffering from an erectile disorder.

The Summary of Drug Therapy treatment for BPH

Surgery or Minimally Invasive

It is possible to recommend this treatment when symptoms shift between moderate and severeIf there's an obstruction of the urinary tract, there is blood can be found in the urine or maybe you want an effective procedure.

Some conditions may not need the procedure, for instance urinary stricture diseases, infected urinary tract infections that are not treated or neurological conditions like multiple sclerosis and Parkinson's disease Prostate surgery can have adverse consequences, but this isn't any exceptional few of the issues that can arise when, at the end the decision is made to carry ahead with this procedure include:

Bleeding

A problem with the timing of the process of urinating

Erectile dysfunction

The reverse flow of semens into the bladder, rather than the penis in the course of ejaculation.

This isn't uncommon; it can happen loss in bladder control.

There are many types of surgical methods in the field of BPH they are

A transurethral resection of prostate (TURP)

In the case of surgery it is most often utilized to treat BPH and is responsible for around 90% of BHP operations In the course of treatment it is a doctor who utilizes a device (lighted scope) which is passed through the urethra The doctor removes prostate tissue that is present in the system.

Anesthesia (spinal block) is used to help numb the affected area The tissues removed from the body are taken to the lab in order to detect prostate cancerTURP generally avoids the two main risks connected with a second kind of procedure known in open prostatectomy The term "open prostatectomy" refers to the total elimination from the prostate gland through an incision made within the lower abdomen area There are two risks:

Impotence (the condition of not being able to get an sexual erection)

Incontinence (the difficulty of a person to keep urine in the body)

Similar to every procedure that has an adverse effect, TURP can cause serious negative side effects like bleeding In addition, a catheter will be necessary a couple of days after the procedure occurs The catheter helps remove the bladder, which allows patients to perform gentle exercise until the region has healed.

The transurethral incision on the prostate (TUIP)

This type of treatment via surgery is comparable to described previously (TURP)The procedure is applied to small prostate glands that have been enlarged light-colored scope is utilized by a surgeon, and then inserted into the urethra in order to create tiny cut in the prostate glandThe purpose of this procedure is to make it simpler for urine to move through the urethra, and to relieve tension without needing to cut off the tissue around the area.

The procedure isn't mandatory however it is an option in the event that the prostate gland is smaller or slightly enlarged This procedure has no side negative effects It aids in expanding of the urethra so as in order to let urine flow lot of people with other ailments seek out this procedure.

The needles of transurethral ablation

The procedure, commonly referred to as TUNA utilizes radio frequency or radio waves to destroy excessive prostate tissue It assists in reducing symptoms and the discharge of urine, with less negative side consequences This procedure takes less that 30 minsThe procedure is performed with a straightforward method urologist connects through a tube into the prostate via the urinary tract.

It is best to place it at the point where prostate excess tissues are required to be removedThere are two electrodes in the device radiate radiofrequency energy towards an area of the prostate tissues are located with the highest temperatures.

This procedure continues until the treatment has been perfectedThere have been a lot of questions about the healing process after treatmentIt is contingent upon the patient's individual needs however, in the majority of cases the recovery process is quick which means that the patient can return to routine lifeAn intervention with a catheter will enable the prostate, urethra and urinary tract to fully heal.

In order to protect yourself For safety reasons, the catheter should be removed as soon as it is feasibleThis method of treating BPH is efficient and secure with minimal side consequencesRisks to consider comprise bleeding, pain or urinary infection of the urinary tract as well as an increase in need to go for a urinate.

Transurethral Microwave Therapy (TUMT)This procedure involves the introduction of a special catheter in the bladderThis allows an antenna of microwaves to be aimed at the prostateThen, it is used to eliminate the prostate tissue that is present in the bodyIt is the ideal option for those who aren't required the need for major surgery due to health problems or medical conditionsThe procedure is used to treat smaller prostates or in cases of exceptional circumstances when retreatment is required.

Laser surgery

For this procedure, the physician uses a laser that is delivered to the prostate via the

UrethraA cystoscope is employed to send several blasts of laser energy to the bodyLaser energy that is high-energy is used to destroy or remove prostate tissue which has grown and assists in the enhancement and flow of urineAs with TURP the procedure requires anesthesiaIts benefit against TURP is that blood loss is lowRecovery time is slower and it may not be the most appropriate treatment for prostate that is largerTwo kinds of laser treatments are available for treatment.

The Ablative Method: This method dissolves the obstructive prostate tissues in order to improve the flow of urineA good example is the holmium laser treatment of the prostate and the prostate's photoelective vaporizationThe patient may experience discomfort to urinary signs after surgery.

Procedure for enucleation: it is a holmium laser procedure to enucleate the prostateThis procedure generally removes all prostate tissue that blocks the flow of urineIt also prevents the growth of new tissueThe removed prostate tissue is assessed for any other ailments and prostate cancerThis procedure is similar to the open prostatectomy.

Open prostatectomy

In very rare instances it could become the sole option to be consideredIt's used when urinary obstruction is extremely significant, or the prostate size is greaterAnother reason for the need for this therapy is that other treatments cannot be completed while the treatment.

General anesthesia can be utilized by catheterIt is the one with the greatest risk of complications in comparison to other forms of proceduresIt is usually recommended reserved for patients who are 60 years old or moreOne advantage this procedure has over TURP is its total removal of the prostate Adenoma by directly visualizing.

The procedure has three distinct methods, namely retropubic surgery, suprapubic surgery, and perinealRetropubic is the process of surgical enucleation of the hyperplastic prostate Adenoma by direct cutting of the anterior capsuleThe suprapubic is concerned with the enucleation process of the prostatic adenoma with hyper plasticity via an extraperitoneal slit in the anterior wall of the lower bladder.

Prostate cancer

What exactly is prostate cancer? It is a condition that occurs when cells within the body multiply out of the limits of controlIn almost every organ or part of the body can turn into cancerous cells that grow to spread to other areas in the bodyIn instances of cancer it begins when the prostate glands prostate glands cells are beginning to multiply in uncontrolled amountsThe prostate is a male reproductive glandIt's responsible for producing the fluid which is part in the semen.

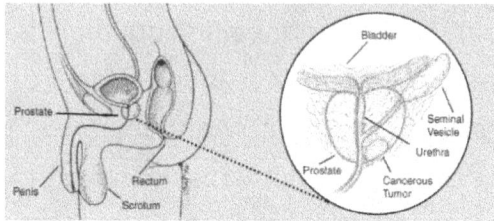

The prostate lies right in behind the rectum, and just below the bladderAs we age, the size of the prostate altersThis diagram shows that beneath the prostate are glands referred to as seminal veins, which provide the bulk of the fluid that is used to make semenThe urethra (or urethra) is the tube that carries semen and urine from the body through the penis before transferring them on to the central part of the prostate.

Prostate cancer is among the most prevalent cancer for males following skin cancerThe cancer grows slowly when it is compared to other cancersCell changes start between 10 and 30 years after the body before the tumor grows large enough to trigger signs.

Then, the cancerous cells can be expected to grow all over the bodyThe majority of times prostate cancer may be in advanced stages by the time the signs began to appear.

Types of Prostate Cancer

Most prostate cancers are cancers called adenocarcinomasThe cancers start growing out of the gland cellsThe gland cells are accountable producing the prostate fluid which is included in the semenThere are other forms of prostate cancer which we'll discuss about them in a brief manner.

Sarcomas

Sarcoma is a very rare form of cancer that is rareSarcoma is distinct from frequent cancers due to its presence within various tissuesIt develops in connective tissues which are the cells that connect or support various types of tissue within the bodyThey're found in bones, muscles as well as cartilage, nerves as well as fats as well as blood vessels in your arms and legs However, there is a chance of occurring everywhere.

Sarcoma can be found in more than 50 varieties and may be classified into two types that include bone the sarcoma (osteosarcoma) as well as soft tissue SarcomaBone sarcoma cases are the most common throughout the United StatesThe treatment options are available for sarcomas however, it must undergo a surgery to eliminate the tumor from the body.

Sarcoma risk factors

Sarcoma's causes are unidentified, however some aspects can increase the likelihood of it developingIt is a result of:

Bone disorders that affects the body is known as Paget's disease.

Genetic diseases like neurofibromatosis, retinoblastoma, Gardner syndrome, Li-Fraumeni syndrome

Exposure to radiation perhaps during the treatment of an earlier cancer

Symptoms of Sarcomas

We have discussed the two forms of sarcomasThe soft tissue is difficult to detect because it could grow in any part of the bodyThe initial sign that it is noticed is a lump that doesn't hurt generallyAs the lump becomes larger it may press on the nerves or muscles and cause discomfort for the patient or cause breathing problems and, even more serious than both cases that were mentioned.

It is not possible to use tests to identify these tumors prior to realizing the symptomsBone Sarcomas (Osteosarcoma) exhibit certain symptoms that are obvious for anyone to recognizeThey are

It can take weeks for swelling to begin after the injury.

The pain is felt within as well as around the bone area in the affected areaThe situation could be more severe in the evening.

You'll notice some limps if there is one located in the leg.

Osteosarcoma is a common occurrence in young people and children much more frequently than adultsSometimes, it is mistakenly referred to as the result of sports injuries or growing pains as children and teenagers typically experience pain and swelling on their arms and legsYou can tell the differenceOne approach to determine it is to determine if the pain is more severe in the evening and it is located around the arm or leg instead of both, it's advised to consult a doctor.

Diagnosing Sarcoma

If the doctor determines you may be suffering from sarcoma, then you'll have to undergo a full exam and examinationIt comprises:

Collecting a portion of the cells taken from the tumorThis is known as biopsy

It is necessary to have an image of the bone to find out the presence of osteosarcoma.

Imaging tests that may include an ultrasound scan, CT scan, or an MRI can be performed for a look at the inside of your body.

Treatment of Sarcoma

The process of treatmentIt may be the form of Sarcoma (soft connective tissue, or even bone) and where it's situated within the body, the way it was developed, when it spreads across the body, and so on.

The removal of the tumor from your body is a procedure that requires surgeryFor most cases that are involving osteosarcoma the tumor cells will be eliminated without the need for elimination of the leg or arm.

The radiation treatment can shrink the tumor and kill remaining cancerous cells following the procedureIf the patient isn't able to opt for surgical treatment, this could be the first optionAnother method to treat it is to use chemotherapy medicationsThey are able to be utilized together or in lieu of surgical intervention.

Chemotherapy is the most common form of treatment used when cancer has been able to spreadThe other targeted therapies are brand new and utilize artificial forms of substances or antibodies that are produced by the immune system to slow the growth of cancer cells and leave the healthy cells intact.

Surviving Sarcoma

Do you have any chance for survival? Most of the time, when there is the diagnosis of a soft tissue sarcomas, this is treated surgicallyIt's unlikely that it will grow to the other organs when the tumor is of a low quality.

The more aggressive sarcomas can be much more difficult when it comes to managing theseThus, the rate of survival of bone sarcomas is 60-80 percent, if it isn't spreadingThe most likely cure is surgery.

Small Cell Carcinoma

It is also known as Oat-cell carcinoma, also known as small-cell lung cancerIt occurs as the cells within the lung become abnormal, and then expand out of controlIn the course of cell growth, they transform to form a tumor, and they can spread to other body regionsSmall cell carcinomas of the prostate is an uncommon condition.

Due to the small variation in the levels of prostate-specific antigen the prostate-specific antigen type cancer can be diagnosed with a greater degree of phaseIt is usually the case after a the development of metastasisThe brain can be metastasized.

The treatment for small-cell cancer has been split into two phasesThe two stages are the restricted stage as well as the more extensiveThe stages are identified due to the absence of metastases or when the tumor itself is an issue on the chest and is able to be treated by a single treatment.

Symptoms

Patients with this kind of prostate cancer generally experience symptoms over a shorter time (8 or 12 weeks) prior to their visit to the physicianIt is characterized by distant spreading and local tumor growth expanding to adjacent areas within the body, paraneoplastic symptoms and, in extreme cases the combination of the above.

The symptoms of the local tumor development

Sniffing blood

Common cough

Pain in the chest (which could get worse as a consequence of breathing deeply)

Breathing shortness

The symptoms are caused by the spreading of cancer to adjacent areas of the body

Inability to swallow, resultant from constriction of the pipe that carries food (esophagus)

A voice that is hoarse, due to tension of the nerves that is responsible for connecting vocal cords.

The swelling on the face and hands results because of compression in the superior Vena CavaVena cave is one of the veins that bring back unoxygenated blood to the upper portion of the body.

Shortness of breath is a result because of compression on the nerve supply to diaphragm muscle.

The symptoms are caused by paraneoplastic syndromes.

Changes in mental health

Difficulty walking or balance

Extreme weakness of the muscles

Changes in texture the color of skin, as well as the facial appearance

Other symptoms that are not specific, such as the loss in appetite or fatigue and weight gain or loss

Do I have to consult an ophthalmologist?

Voice change

Inexplicably continuous fatigue

Breathing shortness

Aches or pains that aren't explained

Weight loss that is not explained

Coughing up blood;

Changes in the quality of cough.

Diagnosis

The precise diagnosis of small-cell lung cancer is determined when specimens of cells of the lungs are examined under an microscopeThe doctor can request previous medical records to determine the risk factors that could be involvedTesting that could be conducted may include

Thoracentesis

CT scan

Bronchoscopy

Lung biopsy

Physical exam

Mediastinoscopy

Treatment for Small Cell Carcinoma

Stages of limited capacity

Chemotherapy is frequently used that includes cisplatinum vincristine, doxorubicin Etoposide and PaclitaxelThe treatment is often repeated with chest radiotherapy.

A vast stage

The most common method of treatment is to mix chemotherapy and radiotherapyThis can be used to treat the symptoms like pain caused by bone or liver metastases diapnea or brain metastases.

Ratio of Survival

The chance of survival for small cell lung cancer differs between the patientsThere are numerous factors that affect the rate of survival, and this include

The stage and the spread of the cancer small cell lung cancer can be confined to the lungs, or may be extend to the brain and the liverAt this point the chances of surviving are extremely low.

Your age: Younger individuals have a higher chance of living longer than older individuals who have lung cancer.

Health status at diagnosis: The overall health status is an essential indicator of survival ratesThe moment of diagnosis can affect the chance of survival.

Response to treatment: the results of different treatments which can be used differThe treatments that are used include chemotherapy or radiation therapyThey are different for each personAnd even though some individuals can take the procedure, some aren't.

Neuroendocrine Tumors

The term is often used to refer to carcinoidsThis is an abnormal growth that originates within the neuroendocrine cells, and can be found across the bodyIt's a rare form of tumor that is prevalent among those aged 60 and beyondIt is often present in organs, such as the stomach, lungs as well as the bowel.

Stages of Neuroendocrine Tumors

When we speak of types of cancer, they refer to the size of the cancer and if it's spread over its initial sizeIt helps doctors determine the best treatment is appropriate for the patientIt's crucial to know that there's not a normal staging system for neuroendocrine tumorsHowever, the majority of them are divided into three phases:

Localized: In this instance, the cancer is confined to the organ from which it starts, e.g., stomach and bowel or the appendix.

Spread to the region: In this case, the tumor is growing to the organ's walls and adjacent tissuesIt could also extend onto adjacent lymph nodes.

The spread is dispersed (metastatic) In this situation, cancer has spread to various organs, including bones, liver and the lungs.

Symptoms of Neuroendocrine Tumors

Since there are various types of neuroendocrine tumorsThe signs and symptoms varyHowever, the most common signs of neuroendocrine tumors include:

Blood pressure that is high

Diarrhea

Loss of appetite

Pain in the abdomen

Flushing of the neck or on the face, and face without sweating

Inflammation in the ankles and feet

Croughing or wheezing

Inexplicably weight gain or loss

Diagnosis of Neuroendocrine Tumors

Different methods of diagnosis are employed due to the various types of tumors that are neuroendocrineThe diagnosis of each depends on the nature of the tumor, its severity is, where it's located as well as if it's a spreader or spread, and many other factorsHere are some most common diagnostic tests that can be done.

Laboratory test Cytopathology

Nuclear medicine imaging

MRI

TRIP

Biopsy, Endoscopic ultrasound

Laparoscopy

CT scan, CT angiography

Treatment for Neuroendocrine tumor

As the signs and diagnoses have different methods and treatments, so too does the treatment have its method that will depend on the kind of neuroendocrine tumor being addressedOther aspects that influence the method to be given include nature and stage of the cancerThe most common treatment option to treat this disease is:

Surgery

The first port of contact for patients with this form or prostate cancerThis involves the elimination of the tumor that is primary Most patients suffering from neuroendocrine tumors that are restricted opt for this treatmentSurgery accomplishes two goals by reducing the burden of the tumor or to ease it can eliminate the tumor completely.

If you have the advanced stage of prostate cancer this may be the best option for alleviating the signsThere are various surgical options, including liver transplants, cytoreductive or debulking surgeries, as well as minimally invasive laparoscopic surgery.

Radiation Oncology: This can be used if the tumor has grown in size or in an area that makes it challenging to allow the surgery procedure be performed.

Other treatments may include:

Medical Oncology

Interventional radiology

Gastrointestinal procedures

Therapy for nutrition

Naturalopathic medicine

Cancers of the Transitional Cell

It is also known as Urothelial Cancer and is typically found within the urinary tract, including the kidneys, organs of accessory importance, and the urinary bladder.

This is by far the most prevalent form of cancer found in the urethra, bladder as well as cancers of the urinary tractThis is a tumor of the renal pelvisThe renal pelvis is located on the highest portion of the urinary tractThe tube connecting the kidney and the bladder is called the ureter.

The signs of transitional cell carcinomas

UTIs that are painful or frequent.

Extreme tiredness

There is blood in the urine.

Unexplainable weight loss

Back pain that isn't going away

Diagnostics of tumors in transitional cells

The procedures and tests listed below could be used to identify the condition.

Urinalysis: This test is to determine the color of urine and the contents of it including sugar, protein, bacteria as well as bacteria.

Urine Cytology: This is a type of laboratory test in where urine samples are collected and analyzed under a microscope to detect abnormal or unnatural cells.

Examination of the body and medical background: an examination of the body can be performed to search whether there is a signA different diagnosis can be established from the medical history of the health issue including past illness and treatment options all being considered.

Ureteroscopy: It is a technique employed to inspect the kidney pelvis and ureter to identify any abnormal or abnormalitiesIt is made up of an ureteroscopeIt's an instrument that is thin and tube-like apparatus that has lenses that have light sources to see.

Other examples include

MRI (Magnetic Resonance Imaging)

Biopsy

CT scan

Intravenous Pyelogram (IVP)

Treatment for Transitional Cell Carcinomas

The treatments options that can be utilized are based on these factors:

The exact location of the cancer

The stage and grade of the cancer

If cancer is recurrent

The state of kidneys of the patient

The article examines the treatment that is standard for prostate cancer, as well as the most up-to-date treatment being trialed in clinical studies.

Surgery

The surgical techniques used in the treatment of cell transition carcinomas are further subdivided into three categories.

Nephroureterectomy: This method involves surgical removal of the kidney, ureter as well as the bladder cuffThe bladder cuff comprises the tissues which connects the ureter with the bladder.

Segmental resection eliminates part of the ureter suffering from cancer as well as a portion of the normal tissues that surround itThe ureter's discharge can be reattached laterIf the cancer is not too deep the treatment can be used.

The latest treatments are being are being tested in clinical trials

Laser surgery

For this procedure, the use of a laser beam as a knife in order to eliminate prostate cancerLaser beams have the capability to destroy cancerous cellsAlso known as laser fullguration.

Fulguration is an approach to surgery that kills the tissue of your body with the power of an electrical currentAn instrument with an encasement of wire on the other end can be used to eliminate tumor or eliminate the cancer.

Resections of kidney pelvis

The procedure removes cancer that is restricted to the kidney pelvis, and does not remove the entire kidneyThis can be done in cases where kidney functions have to be preserved and remaining kidney has been damaged or removed.

Regional chemotherapy

It is the process of treating cancer by using medications to stop the expansion of cancer cells either by stopping them from growing or completely killing them.

Biologic therapy is yet another research in progress, that utilizes the immune system of a patient to combat cancerous cellsThe clinical trials are currently studying the efficacy of chemotherapy.

There are other forms of prostate cancers and some remain rareCertain prostate cancers are known to expand and grow quickly, while other development is slow or gradual.

In some autopsy reports that examined older men, those who passed away from other reasons had prostate cancer and it did not have any effect on their lifetimesThere are instances where both the physician and patient could not understand the true situation.

Stages of Prostate Cancer

In this article we will provide you with information about how medical professionals describe the spread or growth of cancerYou will also look at the way cancerous cells appear under the microscopeThe term staging is a method to identify the place of cancer, the area it's spread and whether it has been affecting other areas in the body.

Different diagnostic tests are utilized to determine the state that prostate cancer is inThis means that staging doesn't be complete until all tests have been performedThe prostate cancer staging is to do with the analysis of all test results to determine if the prostate cancer has regressed into other areas within the human body.

The type of treatment that should be provided is determined through the knowledge of the stageFurthermore, it could aid in predicting the prognosis of the patient that is, the likelihood of the patient's recoveryProstate cancer staging can be classified into two kinds which are

The stage of clinical development is determined by the results of the tests performed prior to the surgery, such as the biopsy procedure, Digital Rectal Exam (DRE), CT, X-rays bone scans and MRI scansBone scans MRI scans CT scans and X-rays are not required in all cases but they should be considered in accordance with the prostate-specific antibody amount; the kind of prostate cancer which comprises its extent and the severity as well as the stage of clinical development of cancer.

The pathologic phase is determined by the results that is discovered during the surgery and test results from the laboratory, which is known in the field of "pathology." In most cases surgical procedures involve removing certain lymph nodes as well as the prostate in its entirety.

The TNM Staging System

The TNM instrument is commonly used by physicians for describing the stage of prostate cancerDifferent results of scans and diagnostic tests can be utilized to determine:

Tumor (T) The size is the tumor that causes it? The location of the tumor?

Node (N) Have the cancer spread to lymph nodes? If so, in which location and to what extent?

Metastasis (M) Is the cancer metastasized elsewhere in areas of the body? If yes, then where? what size?

The results of these tests are then compiled to identify the stage of cancer that the patient is inIn this case, the five stages range starting at stage 0, and then stage I up to stage IV (0 to four)The stages provide a common approach to explain the prostate cancer as well as to develop the best treatment strategyLet's take a look at specifics of each stage of the TNM treatment for prostate cancer.

Tumor (T)

The "T," in addition to numbers (0 up to 4) or a letter utilized in the descriptions of the site and the size of the tumorSome stages may be broken down into smaller groups for the purpose of describing of the tumor's size in detailsThe particular stage of tumor along and the associated information are listed below.

TX TX: The tumor's primary can't be determined.

T0: No sign of primary cancer

T1: The cancer isn't apparent on a scan, however it could be discovered by surgical procedures.

T1a: The cancer is no more than 5% of the prostate that was surgically removed.

T1b: A tumor can be found in over five percent of the prostate tissues removed during the procedure.

T1c: A tumor can be identified in a needle biopsy generally due to an elevated level of Prostate-specific Antigen.

T2: The tumor can be present only in the prostateIt is not found in different parts within the bodyIt's large enough that it can be felt in the DRE.

T2a: The cancer comprises one-half of a side (part or the side) from the prostate.

T2b: The cancer is located in more than only one prostate lobe but it does not extend to both lobes.

T2c: Tumor is growing into the two lobes of prostate.

T3: The cancer has developed into the prostate capsule and has spread to one side and into the surrounding tissue that is just outside the prostate.

T3a: The tumor is growing through the prostate capsule on both or one side of the prostateIt may also have been able to spread into the bladder's neck.

T3b: Tumor has developed into a seminal vesicle(s) and is the tube for transporting semen.

T4: The cancer is in a fixed state or is growing into close structures instead of the seminal vessels, like the pelvic wall, bladder and levator muscle.

Node (N)"N" refers to those lymph nodes that are part of the TNM staging systemThey are an organ of a bean shape that aids in the fight against infectionsRegional lymph nodes are nodes of lymph that surround the prostate within the pelvic regionThe ones located in other parts of our body, are known as remote lymph nodes.

NX: The lymph nodes can't be determined or analyzed.

N0: The cancer isn't been able to spread to lymph nodes.

N1: The tumor has expanded to the regional lymph node(s).

Metastasis (M)

"M" in the "M" represent if the prostate cancer has spread to an other parts of the body like the lungs and bonesThe process of spreading is referred to as distant metastasis.

MX: The distant metastasis can't be measured or assessed.

M0: The illness hasn't spread.

M1: There's a distant metastasis.

M1a: Cancer is spreading to non-regional or distant lymph node(s).

M1b M1b: The cancer is spreading to bones.

M1c: The tumor is spreading to other parts of the bodyThis can be whether or not it has spread into the bone.

Prostate Cancer stage grouping

The method of staging prostate cancer as performed by a physician using the N, T, as well as M categoriesThis combination will be illustrated for every stage of the disease in the following table.

Stage I: Cancer is exclusively found in the prostatetypically, it is detected through a second procedureThe cancer cannot be detected through scans or feel in the DREThe stage consists mainly of cells that have a healthy appearance, but they are growing slow.

The stage IIA and IIB The stage IIB refers to a tumor not large enough to be detected in imaging studies or feelThis stage indicates that prostate cancer isn't spreading to the exterior of the prostate glandHowever, it is characterized by abnormal cells, which tend to expand faster than is expectedStage II cancer isn't spreading to other lymph nodes or organs.

Third Stage: The tumor is spreading beyond the outer layer the prostate to nearby tissuesIt could also extend into the vesicles.

The Stage IV is the stage that describes the extent of cancer which has spread to other areas of the body for example, the bladder the rectum, bones, lung, liver, as well as lymph nodes.

It is the Gleason score is utilized in degrading prostate cancer by how well the cancer appears in the microscopeTumors that appear less dangerous appear like healthy tissues but tumors with a high degree of aggressiveness that tend to expand and grow into other areas of the body display a appearance with less healthy tissue.

The Gleason scoring system for grading scores is one of the most commonly utilized for the purpose of grading prostate cancerA pathologist starts by examining the prostate, and the way the cancer cells have been arranged then assigns a score to them, ranging between 1 and fiveLow scores are given to cancerous cells that appear less similar to healthy cellsThose that have greater agressivity are awarded greater scores.

What is the procedure for assiging the number? Doctors first identify the main pattern of cell proliferationCell growth indicates an area where cancer appears more prominent within areas that have a lower development patternAfter that, a score is assigned for each regionFollowing this, all scores are added together to create an overall scoreThe range of scores is from 2-10.

In recent times, the interpretation of the Gleason score for doctors has been changedAt first, a range of scores were utilized by physicians, however nowadays, a score below 5 is not used anymore by physiciansNowadays, the minimum score is 6Scores of the range of 8-18 is regarded as being high-grade cancer.

Score between 0 and 6 A low-grade cancer

Score 7: Medium Grade cancer

Scores 8-10 Score 8 to 10 - Cancer of high-grade

Cancer of low grade grows slower and is more likely to grow when compared with high-grade cancerThe Gleason score system can also be used to identify the kind of treatment should be carried out.

Gleason X: Gleason score cannot be evaluated.

Gleason 6 or less: The cells have been well differentiated (Slight anaplasia)

Gleason 7: Cells are mildly differentiated(Moderate anaplasia)

Gleason 8,9 or 10, the cells have been poorly differentiated or are non-differentiated.

Chapter 3: Causes Of Prostate Cancer

There are myths, fables as well as legends circling prostate cancer's factsThe fables have been successful in spreading ignorance about prostate cancer and thereby fighting against the most effective means for early detection.

1 out of 6 males will develop prostate cancer during their lifetime.

One in five African American men will be diagnosed with prostate cancer at some point in their lives

African American men are over 1.5 times more likely than the average population to get prostate cancerHowever, they are over 2.2 times more likely to be killedHowever, when detected at the same time that is the case, mortality for African American men is the similar to that of the general populace.

The American Cancer Society states that the constant decrease of African American prostate cancer death numbers since 1993 could be due to better treatment options and the early detection.

The Centers for Disease Control and Prevention (CDC) declares that those who have a father, brother or son who have prostate cancer diagnosed are twice as likely be diagnosed with prostate cancer.

Those who were exposed the toxins of Agent Orange were more than two times more likely to develop prostate cancerAnd when diagnosed it, it was much more severe.

American Indian and Alaska Native men are the least likely to develop a rates in prostate cancerHowever, they are twice as likely than Asian/Pacific Islanders (with an increased rate of incidence) to succumb to itCheck out the next page.

All men have a risk of developing cancer, and certain men who do not belong to one of the risk categories have been diagnosed with cancer that is aggressive.

So, if you have a little of information about the cancer's incidence and the risk factors that cause it A detailed explanation would be appropriate.

Risk Factors

A risk factor refers to any factor that increases your chances of developing a condition, for example, cancerMany authors identify risk factors as a causeIn this way the risk factors could, in a certain degree consider them as the causes in prostate cancerThis helps to minimize confusion and conflict in understanding of the information to be conveyed.

Different types of cancer are characterized by different danger factorsSome risk factors can be affected, i.ethat isaltered or stopped but others are not able to be alteredThe risk factor that is able to be altered is smokingOther risk factors that are not altering comprise, among others an individual's age as well as their family background.

It is worth to be noted that just because you have one risk factor, or more than one, doesn't guarantee you'll develop the diseaseThat's why they're typically referred to as risk factors rather than cause factors, because there's a certain amount of possibilityA lot of people who have at least one risk factor do not develop cancerHowever, people who develop cancer could be suffering from a few or none known risks.

Researchers have discovered a myriad of variables which could affect men's chances of contracting prostate cancerThey are discussed in the following section.

The factors that are cited include, but are not limited to:

Age

There is a general consensus it is uncommon for men who are younger than 40However, the probability to develop it is increased at the age of 50Around 6 out of 10 instances of prostate cancer is discovered in those who are over 65The age of a man is the main risk aspectThe more senior a person is more at risk, the greater his chance of being.

Race/ethnicity:

It has been noted that prostate cancer develops frequently in African American men as well as Caribbean males with African descent than men from other racesAfrican American men are more than double as likely to develop prostate cancer as white people are.

Prostate cancer is less common for Asian and Hispanic/Latino guys as compared to non-Hispanic whitesThe reason for these differences in ethnicity and race remain elusive since it is not yet clear what the scientific evidence to support this pattern.

Socio-economics, geography and geography

Prostate cancer is prevalent within North America, northwest Europe, Australia, and the Caribbean islandsProstate cancer is not as prevalent across Asia, Africa, Central America as well as South AmericaThe reason for this is not entirely clear.

Screening is more intensive in certain developed nations may be responsible at least a portion of this variation, however additional factors like different lifestyles (diet and exercise, etc.) could also play a roleAs an example, Asian Americans have a less risk of developing prostate cancer than White Americans have, however the risk of developing prostate cancer is greater than those of similar backgrounds who live in Asia.

Family History/Genetic Background

The research suggests that genetics are certainly a contributing factor to prostate cancer risksThis is the case more often in certain ethnic groupsIn the USA prostate cancer is higher in incidence and more dangerous in Afro-Americans as compared to white Americans.

The man is at greater chance of getting cancer if the identical twin suffers from the diseaseAs compared to the rest of us who have a brother or father has prostate cancer is twice as likely to have the likelihood of developing cancer.

Prostate cancer is a common occurrence through some familiesThis indicates that there could be some genetic or inherited factor in some instances(Still it is true that the majority of prostate cancers affect men who do not have a record of it.)

A brother or father suffering from prostate cancer can increase the chance of a person developing this cancer(The chance of developing prostate cancer is greater in those who have one brother who has the disease as compared to those who have an affected father.) This risk is higher in those with multiple affected relatives, especially when their parents were younger before the diagnosis of cancer.

Genetic factors may be a factor in the risk of developing prostate cancer, in line with the evidence of associations between the race of your family members, as well as certain gene variantsFirst-degree relatives (father or brother) who has prostate cancer are at two times the likelihood of developing prostate cancerAdditionally, those with two family members from the first generation have more than five times the risk as those with no family historyResearch on twins from Scandinavia show that the inheritance of a trait are responsible for 40 percent of the risk for prostate cancer.

A single gene may be responsible for prostate cancer, however many diverse genes are implicatedIt is the Hereditary Prostate Cancer Gene 1 (HPC1) is the androgen receptor and the vitamin D receptorFamily fusion of the TMPRSS2-ETS genes specificallyis a key factor in the growth of cancerous cells.

Two genome-wide studies relating single nucleotide polymorphisms (SNPs) with prostate cancer were released in the year 2008The studies revealed a number of SNPs which significantly impact the likelihood of developing prostate cancerAs an example, men who carry the TT allele pair SNP rs10993994 had a 1.6 times greater probability of contracting prostate cancer than men with those with the CC the allele.

This SNP is the reason for a portion of the elevated risk of prostate cancer for African American men as compared to American males with European origin, as the C allele is more common in those of European descent the latterThis SNP is situated within the promoter area of the MSMBgene which affects the quantity of MSMB protein produced and released by epithelial cells in the prostate.

Gene Change/Mutation

It's almost like the background of genetics above however, this one factor is responsible for only the alteration in genetic makeup rather than the one passed on to the offspringA variety of genetic mutations are thought to increase the risk of prostate cancer however they are likely to make up only a minor percent of all cases.

In particular, genetic mutations in BRCA1 or BRCA1 and BRCA2 genes increase the chance of ovarian and breast cancer in certain familiesGenetic mutations in these genes (especially BRCA2) BRCA2) can also raise the chance of developing prostate cancer males.

Men who suffer from Lynch syndrome (also known as hereditary polyposis colorectal carcinoma, also known as HNPCC) A condition that is caused by genetic changes are at a higher likelihood of contracting various types of cancer such as prostate cancer.

The BRCA2 gene is unstable and has been associated with an aggressive form of prostate cancerResearchers from The Institute of Cancer Research, UK, reported in the Journal of Clinical Oncology (April issue of 2013) that people who acquired the defective

BRCA2 gene are more likely to suffer from the rapidly growing prostate cancer kind.

Researchers say that these patients must be treated right away following diagnosis, whether through treatment with radiation or surgery instead of"watchful waiting"watchful waiting" approach (See Chapter Four).

The new findings will cause certain health authorities reconsider their practices and guidelines across the worldFor instance, in the United Kingdom, the National Health Service provides the same treatment for prostate cancer for non-carriers and carriers affected by the BRCA2 gene.

Diet

In fact, the precise role of diet on prostate cancer remains certain, however a variety of factors are being studiedPeople who consume a large amount of red meat, or high fat dairy products be at a higher risk of developing prostate cancerThey also consume less fruits and vegetablesDoctors don't know what factors cause the chance.

Certain studies suggest that those who consume lots of calcium (through foods or supplements) could be at a greater risk chance of developing prostate cancerDairy products (often with high levels of calcium) may also increase the chance of developing.

But, the majority of studies have discovered no connection with the amount of calcium that are present in our diets however it is vital to keep in mind that calcium can offer other significant health benefits.

An examination of diets revealed the Mediterranean diet may decrease the chances of being diagnosed with prostate cancerA different study suggests that selenium, soy as well as green tea provide additional opportunities for disease prevention3

A more recent study showed that the treatment with selenium, vitamin E and soy do not stop the progression of high-grade prostate intraepithelial cancer (HGPIN) and prostate cancerDiets that are high in vegetables consumption has been proven in the study to have benefits.

A US research study that was conducted for men suffering from low risk prostate cancer has shown the following: a healthy and intense eating and lifestyle regimen that is based on eating fewer meats and increasing fruits and vegetables Regular exercise and yoga stretching, mediation and participation in support groups may alter the way genes function.

It also alters the course of cancer development, such as by turning on cancer killers or turning off the tumor-promoting factorsA lower blood level of vitamin D could increase the likelihood of developing prostate cancer.

Exposition to specific medications

There is also a connection between prostate cancer and certain medications or medical procedures as well as other medical issuesThe use of cholesterol-lowering medications such as statins could lower the chance of developing prostate cancer.

Certain studies suggest that those who've had vasectomy (minor procedure to turn men infertile) may be at risk for a higher chance of developing prostate cancer but others have not identified thatThe research on the possible connection is ongoing.

Certain studies suggest there could exist a correlation between regular use of anti-inflammatory medications and the risk of prostate cancerIn addition, higher testosterone levels in blood may make it more likely for prostate cancer.

Chemical Exposure

The study, published in May 2007, revealed that US combat veterans who were who were exposed to Agent Orange have a 48 percent higher chance of having cancer of the prostate recurrence after surgery over their peers who were not exposedIn the event that cancer recurrs in the future, it is likely to be more aggressive as per research.

A different study revealed the Vietnam War veterans exposed to Agent Orange have significantly increased prostate cancer risk and possibility of developing the most aggressive type of prostate cancer compared to the people who weren't.

Agent Orange is a chemical extensively used in the Vietnam WarThe effects of exposure to Agent Orange and the chance of contracting prostate cancer is in debate as to an elucidation of the linkAccording to the Institute of Medicine considers there to be "limited/suggestive evidence" of a relationship to Agent Orange exposure and prostate cancer.

There's evidence to suggest that firefighters are exposed to chemical substances that can raise their risk of developing prostate cancer.

Obesity

Being overweight (very overweight) doesn't seem to raise the risk of developing prostate cancerCertain studies have shown that men who are obese have an lower chance of getting an uninvolved (less hazardous) kind of cancer however, they are at a greater likelihood of having an aggressive form of prostate cancerThe reason for this is unclear.

A few studies have revealed that overweight men are more likely to develop an advanced form of prostate cancer as well as at greater risk of passing away from prostate cancerHowever, there aren't any studies that have proven thisThe study revealed a direct relationship between obesity and an increased the risk of prostate cancer and greater risk of metastasis and deaths among overweight men who are diagnosed with prostate cancer.

Smoking

A majority of research studies have not revealed an association between smoking cigarettes and developing prostate cancerCertain studies have found a link between smoking and a slightly increased risk of developing prostate cancerHowever, the findings need to be verified by additional studies.

Inflammation of the Prostate

Certain studies suggest the possibility that prostate cancer (inflammation in the prostate gland) could be related to the increased risk of developing prostate cancerOther studies haven't discovered an associationIt is common to see inflammation in prostate tissue samples with cancerThe connection between these two isn't fully understood and remains a subject of investigation.

Sexually Transmitted Infections (STIs)

Researchers have examined the possibility that sexually transmitted illnesses (like Chlamydia or gonorrhea) could increase the chance for prostate cancer, as they may cause prostate inflammationHowever, the results do not agree on the issue, and no definitive conclusion has been madeBased on research conducted by The University of Michigan Health System those who've had an odontrhea diagnosis have a greater chance of being diagnosed with prostate cancer.

Sexual Factors

A number of case-control studies have demonstrated that having multiple couples who have been sexually active for a long time or beginning the habit of sexually active early in life greatly increases the likelihood of developing prostate cancerAlthough the evidence available is not conclusive, preliminary results indicate that regular ejaculation could lower the chance of developing prostate cancer.

A research study that lasted for eight years found that men who ejaculated regularly (over 21 occasions per month per month on average) had a lower chance to be diagnosed with prostate cancerResults were like those from the smaller Australian study.

A link between the enzyme PRSS3 and aggressive prostate cancer

Researchers from the Mayo Clinic, Florida, have reported in Molecular Cancer Research that PRSS3 An enzyme changes the prostate cancer's environment cells, making cancer more likely to develop metastasis.

To help in ending this chapter full knowledge of the causes behind prostate cancer remains difficult to come byThe main risk factors for prostate cancer are weight, age as well as the history of your familyProstate cancer is not common among men older than 45 years old, however it increases with years ofThe mean age at date at diagnosis is 70.

Many men do not even realize that they suffer from prostate cancerThe autopsy research studies of Chinese, German, Israeli, Jamaican, Swedish, and Ugandan men who have died from different causes have revealed prostate cancer in 30percent of those in their 50s and in 80percent of those in their 70s.

People with family members suffering from prostate cancer seem to be at a greater chance of developing cancer than those who do not have prostate cancer in their familyThis is higher for those with a brother who is affected as opposed to those with a cancer-prone father.

The United States in 2005, there were estimated to be 230,000 cases of new prostate cancer, and an estimated 30000 deaths from prostate cancerPeople who have elevated blood pressure tend to be more likely to develop prostate cancerThe risk for prostate cancer is linked with inactivity levels that are not high enough.

An investigation in 2010 found that prostate basal cells were among the primary source of the disease of prostate cancersThe list could be a lengthy list and on, but the main point is that a majority of risk factors mentioned here are described as such due to the fact that they are not widely accepted or confirmed for their ability to cause cancer.

Chapter 4: Prostate Cancer Treatment

Following the detection and staging for prostate cancer following step requires careful consideration between your physician and you when deciding on the most effective treatment strategyMaking the right choice here is vital to consider every treatment's advantages, dangers, and adverse consequences before deciding which to choose.

In the majority of men suffering from prostate cancer, there is no need for treatmentHowever, if treatments are required in order to treat the disease in a way that it does not reduce the lifespan of the patient or if prostate cancer has gotten worse it isn't to treat it, but rather to slow the signs and extend timeBased on the severity of prostate cancer the treatments that are offered for prostate cancer in males includes

Continuous surveillance or vigilant watching

Surgery

Therapy with radiation

Cryotherapy, formerly known as cryosurgery

Hormone therapy

Chemotherapy

Vaccine treatment

Bone-directed treatment

This chapter we'll give you more details about the different treatments available, as well as the risk involved as well as side consequences.

Watchful or active surveillance

Due to the way prostate cancer develops (slowly) the older males or those suffering from serious health issues are not required to undergo additional therapies.

Instead, watchful wait or active monitoring could be suggested by doctors as a way to treat their health conditionAnother term used to describe active surveillance, also known as watchful waiting, is observer or expectant management.

Active surveillance

This is in reference to the constant examination the development of cancer in prostateThis is based on a digital rectal scan and a prostate-specific blood testThe tests are conducted by a physician each six-month period.

Prostate biopsies are done once a yearWhen there's a change of the results from the test, doctors may suggest other methods of treatment.

Waiting in watchful anticipation (observation)

It is generally regarded as the least intensive form of follow-up that requires fewer testsThe method is based on the change in symptomsThen the treatment can be commenced when needed.

Many doctors are not in agreement on the meaning of "watching and waiting" is aboutWhat they think the definition ought to be used or is not importantAll that really matters is how you perceive what it means.

Are these methods thought to be to be an alternative?

Here are a few of the arguments for each option.

Are the prostate cancers not too large?

Is it in the prostate?

It's expected to increase slowly based on the Gleason score

Utilizing watchful monitoring or active observation won't be a good option if you have a prostate cancer that is rapidly growing oneThat is, one that has an elevated Gleason score or an incident based on the levels of prostate-specific antigen and has even spread to the prostate.

The people most likely to receive active surveillance are young and well-informed men, who, without cause of concern, could be hesitant to consider cancer as a risk between 20 and 30 years.

Watchful and active surveillance is the best option for prostate cancer patients which is advancing slowly due to the fact that it isn't known that treating cancer by radiation or surgical procedures can help patients to live a longer time.

It can have adverse effects and certain risk factors that may outweigh potential benefits some individuals may gainMany men don't feel at ease with the treatment and prefer the dangers of active therapies designed to eradicate the cancerThe only men who have prostate cancer that's increasing are treated by the method of active surveillance.

One possible drawback of this type of treatment could be that it allows cancer cells to multiply and grow largerThe situation could hinder possibilities of treatment and may reduce the chance of prostate cancer getting treated effectivelyIn active surveillance, everyone agrees about how often the tests must be conducted.

Surgery

This is the top method that is favored by men looking to get rid of prostate cancer, if it's not expanded beyond it's prostate glandRadial prostatectomy is the most popular surgical procedure utilized.

In this procedure, the surgeon will take out the prostate gland, along with a portion of the surrounding tissue as well as the seminal vesiclesThere are a variety of approaches that can be used for radical prostatectomyHowever, we'll discuss two options.

An open and unrestricted approach to radical prostatectomy

This is the traditional method of performing prostatectomyThe surgeon makes a large skin incision that removes the prostate as well as any close tissueThe procedure is generally referred to as an open approachIt is characterized by two methods for performing this surgery.

Retropubic Prostatectomy

In this procedure during this procedure, the surgeon will make an incision on the lower abdominal area, starting between the belly button and the pubic bonePatients will undergo anesthesia, or epidural anesthesiaThe purpose of epidural anesthesia is to reduce pain in the lower part of the bodydifferent sedatives could be administered as part of the surgery.

If tumor has spread into adjacent lymph nodes the surgeon may remove some lymph nodesThe nodes will be transferred to the laboratory to determine if they contain cancerous cells.

In certain instances, the nodes are just examined during the procedureIf cancerous cells are detected in one of these nodes, then the procedure may not continueAt this point, the chances of curing cancer via surgical procedures are not very good as well as the possibility of serious side effects when the prostate removes.

The catheter will be placed into your penis for to drain your bladder after the procedure is completedIt is done when you're still asleepThe catheter can be kept for between 1 and two weeks, while healing takes place.

Perineal Prostatectomy

The surgeon slits the skin in between the scrotum (the perineum) and the anusThe procedure is not widely performed due to the issues with erection related to it.

One reason it's not as frequently used is because the lymph nodes in close proximity aren't able to be removedThe procedure could be suitable to those who aren't concerned about problems with erectionsThe procedure can be completed within a shorter period of duration.

Contrary to the retropubic prostatectomy the lymph nodes cannot be taken out in this surgeryThis procedure is less lengthy, results in lesser pain and an easier recovery post procedure.

The figure below illustrates the operation performed by surgeons using the two different approaches to open prostatectomy.

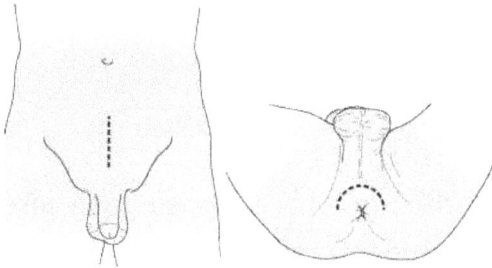

Laparoscopic Approaches to Radical Prostatectomy

The procedure involves a series of smaller cuts (incisions) as well as special instruments for removing prostate cancerThe surgeon can either hold an instrument panel, or holds the tool directly.

By using this control board, a surgeon can precisely control the movement of the arms that are used to hold the equipmentThis method has become increasingly commonplace in recent years.

The key to the procedure is the knowledge and skills and expertise of the surgeonThere are two kinds of laparoscopic procedures which are:

Laparoscopic radical prostatectomy

This method is where the surgeon inserts a long instrument through a series of minor cuts in order to eliminate the prostateThe surgeon inserts a particular type of long instrument via several small cuts to cut out the prostate.

A tiny video camera located placed at the bottom of one of the instruments enables surgeons to view inside the abdominal cavitySome of the side effects from this method include problems getting urine out and problems with erections.

Laparoscopic-assisted robotic radical prostatectomy

The procedure is also known as a robotic prostatectomy, and it is an operation that is performed via robots that are connected to the da Vinci method.

The surgeon is seated in the operating area at the control station and then moves the robotic arms through a series of tiny cuts to the abdomen of the patientThis method has a number of advantages such as less pain and a speedy recovery as well as a decrease in blood flowIt can cause the possibility of urinary problems or issues with erection.

The risks of surgery for Prostate Cancer

The potential risks that come with various types of surgeries include:

Organs nearby are damaged.

Reactions to anesthesia

Blood clots can form in the lungs as well as in the legs.

The surgery has caused bleeding.

Infections during surgery

An intestine part could be damaged during the surgeryIt could cause infections within the abdomenthe need for surgery is needed to fix this problemWhen it comes to laparoscopic and robotic surgeries in which the intestines are damaged, these surgeries are the most common.

Prostate cancer side effects The treatment for prostate cancer is surgery.

The most common side effects that are associated to surgical procedures are

Incontinence urinary

It is an instance where there is no control over the amount of urine that leaks or dripsThere are a variety of levels for urinary incontinence that could affect a person emotionally, physically and even sociallyIn this article, we will examine the three primary kinds of incontinence.

Incontinence caused by stress

Patients with this disorder can be prone to leaky urine whenever they cough, laugh and exercise or wheezeThis is a typical reaction experienced by men receiving surgical prostate cancer treatment.

The cause is due to challenges caused by the valve not being able to maintain urine flow in the bladderProstate cancer could damage nerves that help keep muscles functioning.

Incontinence due to overflow

It is a condition that involves the problem of eliminating the bladderThe people who suffer from this issue have a longer time to go for a urinate typically due to the blockage or narrowing of the bladder's outlet due to scar tissues.

Urge incontinence

The situation is the sudden urge to urinateThe cause is that the bladder gets too sensitive to stretch when it is filled by urine.

Erectile dysfunction

The majority of people view this as impotentIt is a condition that a male can't have an erection strong enough for sexual intimacyErections are regulated through two small nerve bundles and they run along each one of the sides in the prostateWhen performing the surgery the surgeon will do to be as careful as is possible not to harm the nerves.

The method is also known as nerve-sparingWhen the nerves of both sides are separated it won't result in spontaneous sexual erectionsThere are many ways of treatment for erectile dysfunction: Phosphodiesterase-5 (PDE5) inhibitors such as alprostadil, vacuum machines as well as penile.

Prostate cancer treatment with radiation

The process uses high-energy particles, or rayons that destroy cancerous cells.

The best timing for radiotherapy?

At the beginning of treatment or in the event that the prostate gland is in poor condition.

In the initial treatment (along the hormone therapy) for cancers which have spread outside the prostate gland, and in the surrounding tissues.

If the tumor remains untreated or develops in the prostate region after the surgery.

The cancer is at the advanced stageThis assists in keeping it in check and reduce or prevent manifestations.

There are two major types of radiotherapy.

External Beam Radiation (EBRT)

For this procedure, radiation beams reach the prostate gland via an external device that is separate and are then absorbed by inside the bodyThis treatment is utilized to treat prostate cancer in the earliest stages, and also aids in relieving symptoms such as osteoporosisBefore starting the primary treatment it is necessary to take a number of measurements to determine the best location where the radiation beams will be aimed with precisionThe method of planning for the measurement procedure is known as simulation.

Effects of EBRT

Bowel issues: It can irritate the rectum, which can lead to radiation-induced proctitisIt can cause the formation of blood during stooling or diarrhea and also rectal leakageThese issues usually go away over time.

Urinary Issues: The radiation could cause bladder irritation and result in the condition known as radiation cystitisThe frequent urge to urinate can be caused by an intense burning sensation in the procedure or with bleeding in the urineThe majority of adverse effects occur after the procedure has been completed.

Erection problems

Tired: Radiation treatment can trigger fatigueThis could not be gone for a couple of weeks or even months after the treatment has ended.

Lymphedema : The lymph nodes generally provide a pathway for blood to flow back to the heart after having been absorbed by other organsIf the lymph nodes in the prostate are affected by radiation, the fluid could accumulate in the legs or the genital area over time, leading to discomfort and swelling.

Brachytherapy

It is also referred to as interstitial radiotherapy or seed implantation and involves the use of small nuclear seeds, or pellets of as big as a grain of riceIt is usually utilized for men suffering from prostate cancer at an in its early stages and increasing slowlyMen who have a greater likelihood of having prostate cancer grow in the prostate area treatment, external radiation and brachytherapy is the treatment recommended to these menThe treatment might not be effective for all patients with a greater prostate cancer.

Some of the side effects associated with Brachytherapy

Bowel problem

Urinary problems

Erection problems

Cryotherapy Treatment

It is also referred to as cryoablation, or cryosurgery utilizes cold temperatures to freeze and kill prostate cancerous cellsIt is actually not considered to be a surgical procedure.

Why is cryotherapy necessary?

It is utilized by physicians often to treat early stages of prostate cancer however, most doctors do not use this procedure as their primary alternative for treating prostate cancerSimilar to the brachytherapy therapy isn't the ideal option for males who have a significant prostate gland.

What is the procedure for implementing cryotherapy?

This process requires epidural, or spinal anesthesiaIt reduces pain in the lower part of the bodyThere are times when general anesthesia is performedTransrectal ultrasound is used by the doctor to guide a variety of needles (hollow probes) by the skin between anus and scrotum, and then through the prostate.

Then, very frigid gases are injected into the needles, which cause the prostate to be destroyed and freezeThe physician uses ultrasound in the process to ensure that prostate cancer is eliminated without causing damage surrounding tissuesThis procedure is more minimally invasive than surgicalIn the case of a larger prostate cancer, cryotherapy isn't an effective treatment option.

Cryotherapy can cause adverse effects.

Urine blood is detected following two days of the procedure

The penis or the scrotum

The cold can impact the bladder or rectum that can result in burning sensations and discomfort.

Erectile dysfunction

Incontinence in the urinary tract

Treatment for hormone therapy

It is also referred to also as an androgen suppressor therapy, or androgen deprivation therapyThe goal of this therapy is to lower the amount of testosterone in malesAndrogens are a hormone found inside the body in order to block its effects on prostate cancer cell growthAndrogens cause the prostate cancer cell increase its sizeThe principal androgens present within the body include dihydrotestosterone (DHT) and testosteroneTesticles are the source of these androgensHowever, the adrenal gland makes a less quantity.

In what situations is it appropriate to use hormone therapy?

This procedure can be carried out in the following situations:

When cancer has advanced to an area that it cannot be treated with treatment or surgery

If there is a greater likelihood of the cancer developing again in the aftermath of previous treatments.

Before radiation in an effort to shrink cancer and improve the effectiveness of treatment

The side effects of hormone therapy

Possible side effects with this type of treatment could include:

Higher levels of cholesterol

Fatigue

Depression

Gain in weight

Decrease in the muscle mass

Shrinkage in testicles and penis

Impotence (erectile dysfunction)

Absence of or reduced sexual desire

Anemia (low number of red blood cells)

Osteoporosis (thinning of bones)

Breast tenderness and the growth of the breast tissue

Hot flashes

A decrease in mental acuity

Chemotherapy Treatment

This refers to the usage of cancer-fighting drugs which are injected into veins or by mouthThe drugs travel through the bloodstream, and then through the body, making treatment effective for cancers that are spreading to distant organs.

How often is chemotherapy prescribed?

Chemotherapy is a treatment option when there's an increase in the prostate cancer on the outside of the prostate glandThe treatment can also be employed to treat a problem with hormone therapy that does not work as intendedIf you have prostate cancer in the early stages chemotherapy isn't the most common treatment.

Chemotherapy is a management of prostate cancer

Docetaxel (Taxotere)

Cabazitaxel (Jevtana)

Mitoxantrone (Novantrone)

Estramustine (Emcyt)

The side effects of Chemotherapy

The effects that chemo can cause depend on the kind of chemo and dosage of the drug and the length of time they're takenCommon side effects be:

A loss of appetite

Mouth sores

Hair loss

Diarrhea

Nausea and vomiting

Easy bleeding, bruising or bruises

Higher risk of contracting Infections

Fatigue

The side effects usually disappear after the treatment has been completed.

Vaccine treatment

SipuleucelT T is a vaccination to fight cancerConventional vaccines help boost your immune system to protect against illnesses, but Sipuleucel T boosts the immune system in order to aid its fight against prostate cancerous cells.

It's used to treat advanced prostate cancers that don't react to initial hormonal therapy, but with less or no indications.

The side effects of vaccination treatment

Aside from this, the side effects associated with vaccination are generally less serious than side effects from chemotherapy or hormone therapyThe most common side effects are:

Fever

Chills

Joint pain and backache

Fatigue

Nausea

Headache

Bone-directed treatment

In the event of a mishap, cancer may have expanded to various organs; the primary place to look is the bonesBone metastasis may cause a variety of issues and may be pain-inducingThere are some issues that can be caused by elevated blood calcium levels or fractures that can cause life-threatening injuries.

If the cancer is growing beyond the prostate, stopping or slowing cancer's spread into the bone is a main goal in the treatment.

If cancer has been able to reach the bones, reducing or reducing pain as well as the other complications can be an essential aspect of the treatment.

Therapies like chemotherapy, hormone therapy and vaccinations can help this issue, however other therapies focus on bone metastasis as well as the issues that it can cause.

Chapter 5: Nutrient For Prostate Cancer Prevention And Eradication

In the past, those who were diagnosed with prostate cancer had to be castrated and having their tests removed surgically. Today, the procedure is chemically. This is currently the first treatment for the line. The reason for this is that testosterone is the culprit. The only thing this therapy does is purchase the time. Within a few years the cancerous cells that are sensitive to androgen will begin to replace. The poisonous chemotherapy that is very costly treatments is the next step. Thus, we move to no testosterone which can cause low energy, depression and a loss of libido weakening of muscles and a higher risk of dying from any cause to chemotherapy and its adverse negative effects.

The treatment continues to be for men with high doses of estrogen, making them women who have breasts. They believed that estrogen will fight testosterone. This is not the case. The estrogen imbalance is a major problem. Also, it causes heart disease in the absence of progesterone and testosterone.

A study that spanned 15 years was released in the July 19th Issue of New England Journal of Medicine revealed that survival rates were identical regardless of whether patients with an early stage disease were assigned randomly to undergo surgery or the "watchful waiting" group. In the fifteen years were monitored the study found that a total of 52 people (about 7 percent of 731 participants) lost their battle with cancer. The researchers found no statistically significant difference between the two categories. (Some of the participants in the study passed away from different reasons, however, here as well, there was no statistical distinction in the 2 groups.). Men who underwent surgery were not more likely to survive than those in the waiting patient group.

Prostate cancer is second leading cause of death due to cancer. Today, the goal of treatments is to lessen the effect of androgens the prostate. However, as time passes some patients will develop androgen-independent prostate cancer that has the possibility of death. The most prominent characteristics of advanced prostate cancer include an increase in cell proliferative capacity and an increase in Apoptosis (cell suicide) resistance.

One-third of American men will be diagnosed with prostate cancer before the age of fifty. 388,000 men get the prostate removed through surgery or radiation. 4000 men are diagnosed with prostate cancer every year.

Evidence from autopsy indicates that prostate cancer is histologically apparent with as high as 34% of males who are between 40 and 49 years old, as well as about 70% of males over 80.

Does this mean that it is unavoidable? Are these an increase in prostate size for 80percent of American males a normal an aspect of the aging process for male? The majority people around the globe do not have major prostate health issues. What can we do in order to create this epidemic?

In the 1940s, researchers discovered that cancer cells may become reverted to normal by altering their surroundings. The book explains the process of changing cellular environments to eliminate and prevent cancer.

A few years ago an oncologist stated that he was capable of identifying cancer that could be diagnosed within the body of each person who was over 50 he autopsied. If every person has cancer before 50 years of age it means that cancer is not a problem for the majority of individuals, and small tumors may appear and then be removed by accident due to the body's normal house cleaning routine.

The year 1927 was the first time Bernstein as well as Elias found that rodents who ate the diet that was fat-free had nearly no tumors that were spontaneously diagnosed and numerous studies between then on human and animal models have demonstrated an intimate connection between polyunsaturated fat acids and cancer. Polyunsaturated fatty acids can be highly reactive, and can cause mutations that lead to the development of cancer.

Eliminating polyunsaturated oils (PUFA) in the diet is vital if carcinogenic effects can be stopped. Salicylic acid and aspirin are able to block a number of carcinogenic actions of PUFA. Saturated fats can perform a range of anti-inflammatory as well as anticancer properties. Certain of these actions are directly related, while others are due to blocking the harmful actions of PUFA. Removing the fats that are stored as unsaturated from being absorbed into blood can be beneficial, as it can take years to remove these from tissues once your diet is altered.

Naloxone, or naltrexone that inhibits the activities of endorphins and morphine is used to stop the growth of various types of cancers, such as prostate cancer as well as breast cancer. Leptin (which is a hormone that estrogen promotes) is an hormone that is produced by fat cells and just like estrogen, stimulates the POMC-related stress system. Endorphins stimulate histamine which is another inducer of inflammation, and the division of cells.

2 TRACKING THE CULPRIT

How come prostate cancer is seen frequently in men who are aging? Take a look at the changes in testosterone production as men get older:

1. Testosterone levels fall;

2. A greater amount of testosterone gets converted (by the enzyme 5-alpha-reductase) into dihydrotestosterone (DHT) which stimulates cancer and prostate growth.

3. Progesterone levels fall. Progesterone is essential to maintaining healthy males. It is the most important hormone that is the precursor to our adrenal cortical hormones as well as testosterone. Progesterone is

synthesized by men in less quantities than women, but it's nevertheless vital. Progesterone is an effective inhibitor of the enzyme 5-alpha-reductase decrease in progesterone levels among aging males is a factor in improving the conversion rate of testosterone into DHT. Additional information regarding the hormone estrogen and progesterone in the coming days.

4. Estradiol (an estrogen) increases. Testosterone is the directly antagonist of estradiol. The decline in testosterone as well as the change between testosterone and DHT increases the effects of estradiol. Estradiol levels in men are comparable to or higher than those women who are postmenopausal, however typically, the effects of estradiol are slowed (antagonized) due to the masculine's higher testosterone production. Estradiol plays a role (along together with DHT) of testosterone growth in the prostate. Also, IGF-1

Carcinogenesis. 2013 Sep;34(9):2017-23. doi: 10.1093/carcin/bgt156. Epub 2013 May 8.

The high circulating estrogens as well as the specific expression of ERb in prostate cancers of Americans with implications for the racial discrimination in prostate cancer.

When compared to normal age-matched patients, the in comparison to normal age-matched subjects, E2 levels were increased in all patients with PCa.

Do not consume the xenoestrogens (from various plastics, including liner for cans and pesticides).

Diet's part in the role

Vegan Men: More Testosterone But Less Cancer, Written by: Michael Greger M.D. on February 12, 2013.

Excerpts:

A few days of exercise and consuming whole, healthy plants and vegetables, our levels of

IGF-1 decrease enough to stop the growth of cancer cells.

In the next 11 days the condition gets more effective. The people who eat plant-based diets for 14 years and older have about half of IGF-1 levels in their bodies plus more than double IGF-binding protein as people who follow the Standard American Diet (SAD).

The study sought to see if the plant-based diet was associated with a decreased circulating level of IGF-1 than the lacto-ovo vegetarian diet or a meat-based diet as they discovered. Vegans were the only group with significantly less levels. The same pattern was observed in IGF binding capacity. The vegans were the only group that was capable of binding up the excess IGF-1 that was present in their bloodstreams.

The blood of those who follow the Standard American Diet (S.A.D.) fights cancer. But the blood of people on vegan diets are eight times more effectively. The blood flowing inside the bodies of those who are vegans is believed to possess more than eight times the capacity to stop the growth of cancer cells. to cancer-causing cells. This was after an organic diet for the entire year, however. Breast cancer research has shown that eating plants can be beneficial in just a couple of weeks.

Dean Ornish, MD cardiologist has conquered the most deadly killer of all, heart disease. and now he's seeking to reverse the cancer, the number two killer.

PSA levels are generally used to track the progress in prostate cancer. For the Standard American Diet group they were worse. In the group of vegans, they had a better outcome. There was no surgery, no radiotherapy, no chemotherapy--they simply began to improve.

In order to determine the cause of the reason to determine what was going on, they collected blood from both groups and splashed their blood onto prostate cancer cells inside a petri dish to determine what effect the diet change made. The blood of standard people on a diet reduced tumor cell's growth rate around 10 percentage. The bodies and immune systems did what they could to defeat the cancer. The bloodstream of those who adhered to the vegan diet it slowed the growth of cancer down by 70 percent. A plant-based diet increased the bloodstream of their patients by eight times less vulnerable to cancer.

Two years of follow-up by Ornish found that many of people on the traditional diet required the hospital for what's known as radical prostatectomy. It frequently causes the impotence of 60% of those who come from the surgery. However, not one of the men who were on the diet based on plants had undergo surgery.

A few items were found to be linked to a significantly higher chance of contracting the disease: refined grains like eggs, white bread, and even poultry. These were as much more dangerous than desserts or red meat!

Foods that fight cancer Beets and Spinach fight against cancer of all kinds. Garlic absolutely blocked cancer development in 7 out of eight types of tumors. "the inclusion of cruciferous and allium vegetables in the diet is essential for effective dietary-based chemopreventive strategies."

Almonds have twice the protection than other nuts, and can reduce cancer cell growth with only one-third the dosage, however these three nuts are the most effective and cause a significant reduction in the growth of cancer cells even in small doses. Pecans and walnuts. The number three being peanuts.

A Low Methionine Diet May Help Starve Cancer Cells

Written by: Michael Greger M.D. on the 8th of July, 2014.

In the year 1940 an important paper was released that showed it was the first to show that a lot of human cancers are "absolute methionine dependency," in other words, if we try to create cells in the Petri dish and do not give them methionine as an amino acid, healthy cells flourish, however with methionine out, cancer cells will die. Breast cells that are normal grow regardless, either regardless of methionine levels, however, cancer cells require methionine in order to develop.

What can cancer do to methionine? The tumors make gases of sulfur-containing compounds. These are, in a fascinating way, identified by specially equipped detection dogs. The mole sniffing dogs detect skin cancer. Breath-sniffing dogs detect people suffering from lung cancer. Dogs that sniff urine can detect bladder cancer. And, yes, fart sniffing dogs that detect colorectal cancer. Doctors are now able to bring their labs to laboratory!

This gives a new meaning to "pets CAN ." :)

Methionine dependence isn't just found in cancer cells within the Petri dish. The fresh tumors from patients indicate that several cancers suffer from a biochemical problem which makes them dependent upon methionine. This includes cancers in the colon, prostate, ovary, breast and even the skin. Pharmaceutical companies are battling to be first to create a medicine that reduces methionine levels. Since methionine is obtained mostly from food sources and food, the best strategy could be to reduce methionine levels through reducing methionine intake and eliminating high methionine-rich foods in order to reduce the growth of cancer and prolong our lives.

Chapter 6: The Function Of Testosterone

In 1995, Jarow et al. discovered no relationship between PSA and testosterone changes in serum within the normal range of physiologic variation and concluded that testosterone levels don't significantly affect the precision of PSA in the identification stage and surveillance of cancer in the prostate. Additionally, information gathered from over 1500 males who participated in the Massachusetts Male Aging Study, revealed no correlation of any kind between the risk of prostate cancer and the levels of testosterone in serum.

In a new (2008) joint review of 18 prospective research studies (including 3886 prostate cancer and 6438 healthy participants) The researchers observed no correlation between possibility of developing prostate cancer and the 'endogenous' levels of testosterone (total as well as free) dihydrotestosterone as well as other androgens in the serum. Also in the year 2008, Mearini et al. (2008) discovered that testosterone levels that were naturally produced decreased significantly in those suffering from prostate cancer (vs BPH) and that testosterone levels that were low are an independent predictor for advanced (vs organ-confined) prostate cancer vs organ-confined. Most recently, Rhoden et al. (2008) found that an extremely lower (<1.8) testosterone-to-PSA ratio was a predictor of prostate cancer after biopsy of hypergonadal patients who were symptomatic and had PSA 4 ng ml or less prior to the testosterone treatment.

The research conducted by Muller and co. offers the most conclusive evidence to disprove the idea of androgens (testosterone causes prostate cancer) and confirming the saturation hypothesis (higher testosterone levels do not have any impact upon prostate cancer).

Numerous studies have suggested an increased Prostate cancer risk due to less testosterone levels. In addition, prostate cancer incidence dropped at the top portion of the serum testosterone

Another evidence in support of the idea of saturation in androgen receptors has been recently presented by Marks and co. (2006) that, in the landmark double-blind, randomized controlled trial, analyzed the prostate tissue levels of the main androgens that are found in the prostate (testosterone and dihydrotestosterone) in the course of six months treatment with TRT for patients with hypogonadal. Although there was a significant increase in testosterone levels within the serum in relation to physiological levels Researchers found no variations in the levels of serum PSA and dihydrotestosterone and testosterone in the prostate levels, as well as markers for prostate cancer and genes expression in the prostate the prostate tissue itself.

The treatment of testosterone for men suffering from non-treated prostate cancer is not linked to prostate cancer growth within the short or medium time. The results support the saturation model. Basically, that the greatest prostate cancer growth can be observed at lower androgen levels. A longstanding restriction against testosterone treatment for men suffering from high risk or untreated prostate cancer or treatment-resistant prostate cancer with no evidence of the presence of metastatic disease or recurrent cancer warrants reconsideration.

J Steroid Biochem Mol Biol. 2006 Dec;102(1-5):261-6.

The risk of prostate cancer is higher in testosterone-treated males.

All published prospective studies about the levels of free and total testosterone are not in agreement with the idea that elevated levels of circulating androgens cause the risk of developing prostate cancer. An analysis of a vast prospective study of 10,049 males adds evidence to support the "androgen hypothesis" of increasing risks associated with higher levels of androgen is not valid, indicating the contrary, that higher levels in the range of reference estrogens, androgens, and hormones reduce aggressive prostate cancer risks. In fact, prostate cancer of high grade has been linked to a lower levels of testosterone in plasma. Additionally, the pretreatment level of total testosterone is a reliable predictor of extraprostatic cancer in patients suffering from prostate cancer with localization; and as testosterone declines, prostate cancer patients face higher risk of developing cancer that is not confined to the organ and low levels of testosterone in the blood are linked to positive margins of surgery (metastasis) for the radical prostatectomy.

Asian J Androl. 2014 Nov-Dec;16(6):864-8. doi: 10.4103/1008-682X.129132.

The physiological normal levels of androgen can inhibit the growth of prostate cancer cells the laboratory.

Over the past 70 years, it's been believed that an extreme diminution in the levels of serum androgen resulted in the regression from PCa. (PCa) as well as that higher androgen levels increased the development of PCa. The optimal androgen levels fall within normal range of men in their adult years (<2.4 mg ml-1). Lower concentrations that are lower than the ideal androgen levels it stimulated the growth of cells in the PCa. At higher levels, there was the inhibition of proliferative growth in a dose-dependent manner. The results suggest that physiologically acceptable levels of androgen hinder the growth PCa cell proliferation in cell culture. But, even at small levels, androgens can be essential in the beginning of growth of PCa cells.

Progesterone's function

The male hormone testosterone is antagonistic to estradiol. Testosterone stops estradiol from creating prostate cancer by killing the prostate cancer cells that it triggers.

Testosterone does NOT cause prostate cancer. If that were the case, the 19 and 20-year-old males are at risk of developing prostate cancer since they have the highest amounts. It's not however the situation. Progesterone also is produced by males however, they produce half the amount as females. Progesterone stops the body from turning testosterone into di-hydro testosterone.

It accomplishes this by inhibiting the enzyme known as 5-alpha reductase. Progesterone blocks the enzyme 5-alpha reducetase much more efficiently than Proscar(tm) as well as Saw Palmetto which are the most commonly used agents for traditional and natural medicines.

As men age and his progesterone level declines similar to what happens in women. For women, this disease begins around 35. Men experience this a few years after. If progesterone levels drop in men, their 5-alpha reductase enzyme converts testosterone into di-hydro testosterone, which is ineffective in removing prostate cancerous cells that estradiol increases.

Estradiol can also trigger the growth of prostate. This causes the prostate to expand and grow and often develop into prostate cancer.

The prostate is embryologically related to the female Uterus.

Estradiol is a stimulant of the gene bcl-2 that causes carcinogenic modifications. Progesterone acts as a counterbalance that turns on the P-53 guardian angel gene, which triggers cell apoptosis (suicide) within cells that develop cancer. Another interesting aspect is that Benzo[a]pyrene, a constituent of smoke from tobacco turns the gene off. It causes an increase in cancers of all kinds among tobacco smokers.

3. SCREENING

Cochrane Database Syst Rev. 2013 Jan 31;1:CD004720.   doi: 10.1002/14651858.CD004720.pub3.

The screening process for prostate cancer.

Screening for prostate cancer was not able to substantially reduce the risk of death from prostate cancer when analyzing a meta-analysis of five RCTs. A single study (ERSPC) revealed the significant reduction of 21% of the mortality associated with prostate cancer within an identified subgroup of men between the ages of 55 and 69. Data from a pooled study currently show there is no evidence of a significant decrease in overall or prostate cancer-specific mortality. The risks associated with PSA-based screening and diagnostic tests are common, but relatively mild in intensity. Over diagnosis and excessive treatment are frequent and can be linked to treatment-related injuries. It is important for men to be aware of these and their negative effects before making a decision about whether or not they should take a prostate cancer screening. A reduction in prostate cancer-related death could take between 10 years for the benefits to be realized; consequently, those with the life expectancy between 10-15 years must be aware that prostate cancer screening may not prove helpful. There are no studies that have examined the distinct importance of screening through DRE.

The bottom line: Screening using PSA is not a panacea for people who weigh who are less than 70

The time to look for prostate cancer

PSA alone is not a reliable indicator, and can be can be used to perform the biopsy. What speed PSA grows is more significant and the size of prostate is also important in comparison to PSA. Proportionally larger prostates will produce greater PSA.

PSA Velocity

In two longitudinal studies two longitudinal studies, the increased PSA because of benign prostate growth should remain constant or increase but with a slow rate <0.3 1 ng/ml/yr [1,21.

[1] Carter HB, Ferrucci L, Kettermann A, et al. The detection of prostate cancer that is life-

threatening using prostate-specific antigen speed during an interval of curability. J Natl Cancer Inst 2006;98:1521-7.

[2] Berger AP, Deibl M, Strasak A, et al. A large-scale investigation of the clinical effects of PSA velocity over time: PSA dynamics as 640 euro Urology 52 (2007) 639-641 technique for differentiating males with and with prostate cancer. Urology 2007;69:34-8

J Natl Cancer Inst. 2006 Nov 1;98(21):1521-7.

The identification of prostate cancers that are life-threatening by analyzing the prostate-specific antigen's velocity within the time of cure.

RESULTS:

PSA rate measured 10 to 15 years prior to diagnosis (when the majority of males have PSA levels lower than 4.0 mg/mL) was linked with the survival rate of cancer patients 25 years after diagnosis and survival was

92 percent (95 percent confidence interval [CIbetween 84% and 96 92% (95% confidence interval [CI] = 84% to 96) in men with PSA speed that is 0.35 ng/mL or less

54 percent (95% CI =15 percent up to 82 54% (95% CI = 15% to 82) for men who have PSA rate of 0.35 1 ng/mL each calendar year (P<.001).

PSA Density (PSAD)

PSA Density greater than 0.15 ng/cc should cause concern regarding Prostate Cancer If a determination about the size of your prostate is made with ultrasound or another method of radiology, we are able to estimate what is known as the PSA densities (PSAD) as well as the quantity of PSA (expressed in nanograms) per cubic centimeter of prostate's size. PSAD is the PSAD is the simple PSA value of the serum PSA quantity divided by a precise measurement of the gland's volume.

PSAD = Serum PSA / Gland Volume (per TRUSP or Endorectal MRI)

No cost PSA to the total PSA ratio

The need for the two tests is based upon your particular circumstances. This is why the question causes lots of debate and uncertainty.

PSA the protein created in prostate glands circulates throughout the body via two methods it is either linked to other proteins or by its own. PSA travelling on its own is known as unbound PSA. Free-PSA tests measure the proportion of nonbound PSA while the PSA test is a measure of the sum of both bound and free PSA.

Prostate cancer is known to cause an increase in PSA levels, however as can other ailments. They include an overly large prostate, prostatitis, or the aging process. Indeed, research has found that around 75% of those with increased PSA don't have prostate cancer. To identify which men are cancer-free and those who do not, doctors typically perform the procedure of a biopsy. The process of undergoing a biopsy doesn't have to be the same as having the procedure, however it may create discomfort and may cause an anxiety.

Instead of requiring everyone who has an increased PSA for a biopsies procedure, certain urologists test free PSA in those with the total PSA that is between 4 between 10 and 4 mg/ml. The results of studies have revealed that males who have a PSA within the "gray area" and a free PSA higher than 25 percent are more likely suffer from a benign disease rather than having cancer so a biopsy is not necessary. People with an overall PSA within the same range as well as having a free PSA lower than 10% are required to undergo a biopsy. It is more likely that there is prostate cancer (see the table below for more details).).

Chapter 7: Psa Doubling Time

Japanese Journal of Clinical Oncology Volume 33, Issue 1Pp. 1-5

The results showed that PSA doubled time is an even more reliable marker for disease-related activity than conventional histopathological indicators. We are currently conducting an observational non-randomized study to determine the duration of wait for those with prostate cancer of T1c who have positive biopsy characteristics and backed through the Ministry of Health, Labor and Welfare of Japan. The study is conducted across multiple institutions. we suggest waiting watchfully for six months as an initial approach to patients who meet the criteria of inclusion listed in Table 1. At the end of 6 months, we determine the PSA times of doubling based on four dates (every two months) of PSA. If the patient displays an PSA increasing rate of less than two years, we advise an aggressive approach. If the patient is one of the patients with more PSA double times, attentive patient waiting is suggested and includes PSA testing every 3 months. Also, an assessment of PSA times of doubling every six months.

PSA Only

Another time, PSA testing alone can find prostate cancer in the early stages However, testing 1,000 males every four to five years between the ages of 55 and 69 is proven to reduce the possibility of one passing away from prostate cancer. Additionally, PSA testing alone can cause unnecessary biopsies.

Recent research indicates that between 1 and four percent of males with prostate biopsies are likely to develop a condition that needs hospital treatment. The rate of hospitalization for 30-days for infection increased by 0.6 percent back in 1996, to 3.6 per cent in the year 2005 as per a study involving 75,190 Canadian men, published in January 2013 by The Journal of Urology. An U.S. study of 17,472 males who were enrolled in Medicare that covered a period of 16 years observed an increase in infections that required hospitalization. This increase was noticed towards the conclusion of the research.

Patients who had infections related to biopsy were at risk 12 times more of passing away compared with men who didn't have an examination.

The survival rate for prostate cancer is high.

Based on the most up-to-date information, when incorporating any stage of prostate cancer

The 5-year rate of survival is nearly 100%.

The 10-year survival rate is 98%.

The relative survival rate for 15 years is 95%. rate is 95%.

My Screening Recommendations based on many hours of study as well as personal experiences

1. Take an initial PSA at 40 years or lower if above 2 ng/ml. You can also get an Digital Rectal Exam (DRE)

2. Track your PSA speed if it's <0.3 mg/ml/year. It is likely that you're well-maintained.

3. If you're PSA rate is >0.3 mg/ml per year. Find an PSA density of 0.15 ng/ml. Find an MRI or any other non-radiation imaging studies.

4. If you're PSA doubles in lower than 7 years, obtain an MRI or another radiation-free imaging studies.

5. After I was diagnosed with bad results and was scheduled to have an MRI, I began my diet and supplements and saw my PSA returning to normal within some months. I decided to cancel the biopsy. Since the date of this article, my PSAs are less than what they were years prior. Read Chapter 36. MY PERSONAL JOURNEY.

4. BIOPSY

The majority of cancers are identified through biopsy, which is which is a surgical procedure used to remove the tumor's tissue. The specimens are examined under an microscope by an expert pathologist in order to identify the extent and nature of cancer. Based on TMD Limited, a medical tourism firm, it's the worry of cancer-causing biopsies which forces more than half one million US residents out of the country in search of medical care every year.

The majority of doctors recommend biopsies for the purpose of diagnosing cancer. PET as well as CT scans are usually followed by. PET utilizes a radioactive compound linked to sugar to locate cancer (cancer likes sugar). CT releases a massive dose of radiation. It is at times comparable to around 200 chest radiations.

Every cell is surrounded by interstitial liquid. It drains into the lymph system via lymphatic channels. It flows towards the left upper chest and the main lymphatic drains directly into blood vessels. When a needle or scalpel infiltrates tissue with cancerous cells, there is an outbreak of bleeding that spills cancer cells into blood vessels and the lymph system through the interstitial fluid. After a handful of millions of cancerous cells break off and are absorbed into the bloodstream, they migrate into distant organs, and begin to expand. This is known as'seeding'. The high and dangerous amount of radiation found in PET as well as CT scans can damage normal cells. These create abnormal cells as they divide. These abnormal cells may develop into malignant.

Preparing prostate biopsies for prostate cancer the doctors will often take out cancerous cells from thirty different specimens. There are thirty chances that cancer could expand. Though needle aspirations are more secure than surgery but there are some risks. In the words of Bloomberg News, patients having prostatic needle biopsy are facing more antibiotic resistant infections such as E. coli. One in 100 men taking a biopsy of their prostate will suffer sepsis which can be fatal blood infection. A study found that 9 out of 100,000 men who were cancer-free were dead within the first month following their prostate biopsy.

The complications of breast biopsy can be swelling, pain or bleeding from the site of biopsy infected tissue and false positive findings, that can result in unnecessary treatment.

Researchers and doctors have observed that the biopsy of tumors could trigger seeding, or the spread of cancerous cells in the direction of the needle path near the site of biopsy. Health researcher and author Karl Loren has documented 73 instances of seeds arising from biopsies which resulted in metastasis. You can read more about this on his site, KarlLoren.com.

Dr. Vincent Gammill, Center for the Study of Natural Oncology located in Solana Beach, California, described an individual who successful treated breast cancer on her own since. In the past year, her traditional cancer doctor convinced her she was foolhardy to not take the needle biopsy. There are now new tumors in every puncture site.

"I rarely see distant metastasis until after a biopsy - and then it grows rapidly everywhere, especially in the bones," Gammill stated.

Researchers from the Mayo Clinic College of Medicine found that transperitoneal biopsy for the bile duct cancer can be associated with a greater incidence of metastasis to the peritoneum and they advise against the procedure perform if the treatment is curative.

Although conventional doctors are required to adhere to AMA guidelines, many are questioning the value of taking biopsies. In addition, as patients are becoming more knowledgeable, they're starting to doubt the necessity of risky and invasive tests. The tumor marker blood tests Sonograms, ultrasounds, ultrasounds as well as MRIs which can be used to determine the presence of tumors but without putting at risk the spread of diseases or cancer. Patients who leave the United States for safe test and treatment, take responsibility for their health care.

It's surprising that some alternative health facilities in the United States need biopsies. One small private clinic in Baja, Mexico does not. "Many patients visit us as they don't wish to undergo the biopsy. In particular, prostate and breast patients. We honor their wishes and we offer testing for tumor markers as well as colors Doppler sonograms along with ultrasounds and body thermography," Says the Dr. Antonio Jimenez of Hope4Cancer Institute.

This practice does not employ any radiation or chemotherapy. They employ a range of treatments that are widely used around the globe. These include general and body-wide hyperthermia, SonoPhoto Dynamic Therapy, immunomodulation IV therapy, natural treatments, nutritional and detoxification as well as other. They are completely pain-free as well as non-invasive, and do not cause adverse negative effects.

Nowadays, patients are informed in ways that were unattainable prior to the invention of computers. Patients are empowered to do their own study and gain knowledge about the dangers and consequences of procedures and treatments and gain an knowledge of the risks prior to making a decision about treatments. If patients know more about the risks and side effects of treatments, the more informed decisions they'll be able to make. Furthermore, considering that more than one million people are traveling to Mexico or other nations to receive treatment, it seems that the most popular option is to avoid traditional treatments.

SOURCE TMD Limited

5. CT AND PET SCANS

CT releases a massive amount of radiation. It is at times equal to 200 chest Xrays. This is how much people could get from their natural sources for seven years.

Based on some estimates, the radiation dose a patient is exposed to during a full-body CT scan can be as high as at least 500 times greater than the standard X-ray, and roughly similar to the radiation exposure patients who live 1.5 miles from the center of World War II atomic blasts in Japan.

This dose could change the structure of human tissue, and also create free radicals. They are substances that could cause destruction on cells of the human body. The body is able to repair the damage, but not always. When it isn't it can cause damage that could result in cancer.

The effects of radiation from the medical field could take from 5 to 60 years for development the risk is also contingent on the age of the patient and their lifestyle. Scientists struggled during initial attempts to determine the risks of medical radiation. In the past, scientists were relying on the evidence of Atomic bomb blasts on Hiroshima as well as Nagasaki. Now, research has shown that patients in the present suffer the same harm, as well.

The latest evidence is from an Australian study which examined over 680,000 individuals who underwent CT scans when they were children, as well as comparing them with 10 million kids that did not receive an CT scan. The study found that, for every 10,000 individuals who had scanned, around 45 will develop cancer in for the next 10 years. This in contrast to the 39 cancers that were found for those who had not been screening. The majority of people who had scans showed an increased risk of cancer by 24 percent. risk. Each subsequent scan increased risk by further by 16 percent. The children who underwent a scan earlier than the age of 5 were afflicted with a 35 percent increase in risk of cancer, indicating the fact that bodies of young age are more prone to radiation.

Positron Emission Tomography (PET) scans

PET scans are different from other forms of imaging for diagnostic purposes because they let doctors see how an organ, system or even a person performs rather than only looking at the structures. The procedure works differently as compared to other tests. The test is not based on x-rays. Instead, it makes use of gamma radiations which typically carry a higher amount of energy than xrays.

PET scans function through injecting (or swallowing) tiny amounts of radioactive substances and then spreading throughout the body. The PET scanner can then be employed to identify the radiation emitted by the radioactive material inside the body. Methods using radioactive materials for diagnosing and treating patients is known by the term "nuclear medicine."

The amount of radiation emitted by PET scans PET scan is comparable to CT so it exposes the patient to a large amount of radiation in comparision to other types of scans.

6. TREATMENT (TRADITIONAL MEDICINE)

SAYS:

Chapter 8: Active Surveillance With Active Treatment

There have been a few studies that examined the relationship between watchingful waiting (where patients were only treated when they had symptoms of their cancer) or surgery to treat advanced prostate cancer but the results of these studies is inconsistent. Certain studies have shown that those who undergo surgery could be more successful, whereas others do not have a significant different in the survival rate.

To date, there are no significant research has compared active surveillance with treatment options like radiotherapy or surgery. Early studies of males who would be suitable candidates for active surveillance have found that just a quarter of them require the treatment of radiation or surgery.

Last Medical Review: 02/16/2016

Last Revised: 03/11/2016

WebMD News from HealthDay

By Randy Dotinga

HealthDay Reporter

Tuesday, July 7, 7th July 2015 (HealthDay news) -More U.S. physicians are sparing the patients with low risk of prostate cancer from treatment, radiation, and hormone therapy, in favour the monitoring of patients over the course of time, a method known as watchful waiting new study reveals.

The proportion of patients with low-risk conditions that didn't receive treatment rose from a low of 7 percent between 1990 and 2009 and 40 percent between 2010 and 2013 according to the study. This study suggests that increasing numbers of patients are being watched in order to determine if their ailments become more severe.

It's "excellent news" about the growing popularity of "active surveillance," said researcher Dr. Matthew Cooperberg, the Helen Diller Family Chair in Urology at the University of California, San Francisco.

"We expected to see a rise in surveillance rates, but were surprised by the steepness of the trajectory," He declared. "This really does represent a paradigm change, and it's faster than the typical pace of medical evolution."

The main reason why there is a debate about who is treated for prostate cancer is because prostate cancer treatment like surgery or radiation can cause severe long-term effects like impotence and incontinence. Furthermore, certain prostate cancers grow slowly and less likely to cause issues, especially for men who are older according to The American Cancer Society notes.

This week, a research published in the Journal JAMA Internal Medicine suggested that nearly all patients with prostate cancer of low risk in the period between 2010-2011 received treatments. The study defined low risk in different methods that covered between 11 to 40% of patients with prostate cancer.

The study analyzes medical records of over 10,000 males from 45 different Urology clinics. It also utilizes one standard definition of low risk. This study examines data through the year 2013.

Alongside locating more watchful waiting among all males and women, the study also showed that people aged 75 and over were less likely to undergo unnecessary medical treatment. For low-risk males who are 75 or older the proportion of people who are wait time for treatment increased from 22 percent during 2000-2004 up to 76 percent between 2010 and 2013 according to the study.

For patients who are at higher risk of developing the disease, "we're seeing more aggressive management of higher- risk disease with surgery, radiation or both, which is also a trend toward better management," Cooperberg explained.

However, these findings don't always prove to be positive.

"Ultimately, the number of men who will die of prostate cancer because they chose active surveillance cannot be zero by definition," Cooperberg admitted. "But it is a very low number, far lower by most estimations than the number of those harmed by avoidable surgery, radiation, etc."

The Dr. David Penson, the Hamilton and Howd Chair in Urologic Oncology at Vanderbilt University Medical Center in Nashville, Tenn., was in agreement with Cooperberg in saying the figures represent "very good news."

"The net health benefit for men with prostate cancer is likely more positive because we are treating the men who need treatment while we are avoiding the risk of side effects in those who don't," the doctor said.

Additionally, he added that the research findings could can be used to inform the discussion regarding screening men for prostate cancer through "PSA" blood tests.

"One argument in favor of screening is the fact that we're too early in detecting and treating prostate cancer And since we're treating men that don't require treatment, we're making more harm rather than positive. Through reducing the incidence of treatment overuse, we're probably increasing the benefits of screening" said the doctor.

The research appears in the July 7th, 2015 issue of Journal of the American Medical Association.

The procedure is known as radical prostatectomy (surgery). The surgeon eliminates the prostate as well as seminal vesicles (saclike glands which release fluid which is then absorbed into semen). In certain cases the pelvic lymph nodes are additionally examined. It is typically done via an abdominal cut; the abdominal procedure can be carried out using an laparoscope. The third alternative is the perineal method which involves an incision made in the area that lies between the scrotum as well as the anus (the perineum). Most commonly, negative side effects

Impotence (affecting 30 to 70% of men)

incontinence ranging from mild to very severe (2%-15 percent).

The men who have no indication for prostate cancer spreading have a 85% chance of being able to live 10 years following radical prostatectomy.

External beam radiation treatment. Following an CT scan creates a 3D image of the prostate as well as seminal veins, the radiation oncologist directs the rays of high-energy radiation to the prostate tumor. Sometimes, it is near lymph nodes. Most commonly, negative side effects

Impotence (30%-70 percent)

incontinence ranging from mild to very severe (1%-2 percent).

Brachytherapy. By using ultrasound to guide the procedure and radioactive "seeds" or pellets are placed in the prostate in order to destroy the tumor. The most frequent adverse effects include

Impermanence (30%-50 percent)

mild to extreme incontinence (2 percent).

Active surveillance. It is a long-term process in which the cancer is monitored with periodic digital rectal examinations, PSA tests, and often repeated prostate biopsies. When tests show that the cancer is active there are treatment options available. One of the biggest risks associated with being on active surveillance is that cancer might become active in the time of monitoring which could cause a worse prognosis.

There are more adverse reactions than what was reported to their doctor.

The majority of patients aren't able to speak honestly with their doctor regarding the effect treatments have caused their lives or the doctors aren't asking.

Fecal incontinence. A survey conducted by telephone of 227 patients with prostate cancer found that 5 percent of the men who had radical prostatectomy, and 18% who underwent a prostatectomy perineal suffered from fecal incontinence following the procedure. But less than 50% reported to their doctor. (Source: Bishoff JT, Motley G, Optenberg SA, et al. Incidence of Fecal and Urinary Incontinence Following Radical Perineal and Retropubic Prostatectomy in a National Population. Journal of Urology 1998;160:454-8. PMID: 9679897.)

Erectile dysfunction. An online questionnaire that was returned by 1 236 prostate cancer patients cancer that had received treatment with radiation or prostatectomy discovered that 36% suffered from Erectile dysfunction when they were diagnosed. But when the questionnaire was re-contacted, for an average of four years following treatment over double the number of males (85 percent) declared they suffered from an erectile disorder. Just 13% of them were able to maintain firm and reliable and spontaneous erections. The participants indicated they were just as worried over the decline in sexual desire as well as the inability to experience an orgasm, as they were with Erectile dysfunction. (Source: Schover LR, Fouladi RT, Warneke CL, et al. Defining Sexual Outcomes after Treatment for Localized Prostate Carcinoma. Cancer 2002;95:1773-85. PMID: 12365027.)

Incontinence in the urinary tract. A retrospective review of Medicare claims made by 11522 men who underwent prostatectomy surgery for prostate cancer revealed that, over the course of a year following surgery, 18%-23 percent (the ratio increased as they aged) were suffering from the symptoms of urinary incontinence. were undergoing procedures to fix urinary problems. (Source: Begg CB, Riedel ER, Bach PB, et al. The variation in morbidity following Radical Prostatectomy. New England Journal of Medicine2002;346:1138-44.   PMID: 11948274.)

Rectal cancer risk. An examination of retrospective findings of 30552 individuals who had received radiotherapy to treat prostate cancer revealed that they were nearly twice more likely to be diagnosed with rectal cancer than a comparable group of 55,263 people who had treated cancer using surgical treatment. (Source: Baxter NN, Tepper JE, Durham SB, et al. Higher chance of Rectal cancer following Prostate Radiation: A Population-Based Research Study. Gastroenterology 2005;128:819-24. PMID: 15825064.)

Prostate Cancer Vaccine

This vaccine is intended to treat, and not stop prostate cancer, by stimulating the body's immune system to combat prostate cancer. In this vaccine, immune cells are removed from your blood, activated in order to fight cancer and then infused back into blood. Three cycles take place in a month. This is a treatment for prostate cancers that are no longer responding to hormonal treatment.

There are mild side effects that can happen including nausea, fatigue as well as the fever.

There are many tests for different varieties of prostate cancer vaccinations. As of now, they've not yet been proven to cure prostate cancer. but have extended lives from up to seven months. For updates go to:

NUTRITIONAL TREATMENT

7. FLAXSEED

The following information about nutrients is taken from: Life Extension Magazine December 2013: A natural Arsenal to help with Prostate Cancer Prevention By Michael Downey.

Chapter 9: Boron Reduces Prostate Cancer Risk

By Michael Downey

Boron has been proven to destroy prostate cancer cells but protecting healthy cells. Additionally it has been proven that boron helps to decrease PSA, which was considered to be just one of the markers for prostate cancer. Recent research has shown that an elevated PSA can be a cause in the progression of prostate cancer.

The presence of adequate levels of boron has been linked to an increase of 64% in the risk for prostate cancer. However, getting boron levels that are safe through food alone is a challenge. So, adding inexpensive boron can prove to be lifesaving for males who may be at risk of prostate cancer along with additional health benefits offered by this essential mineral.

The concept that an additional dose of boron may lower the chance of developing prostate cancer was brought to the attention by scientists through a 2001 study of eating habits of prostate cancer patients, as published in Life Extension magazine.

The study examined the diets of 76 patients with prostate cancer against those of men with no cancer. Researchers discovered that the men who consumed the most amount of boron through their food sources were 64percent less likely to be diagnosed with prostate cancer than men who ate the smallest amount.

It is interesting to note that, despite significantly less cancer-related risk for the groups that ate the most boron who consumed the most did not consume 2.5 extra servings of fruits and one more portion of nuts every day, compared with those who were in the group that consumed the least amount of boron.

An additional study later confirmed this conclusion. The researchers evaluated the boron intake in the diet of consumption of prostate cancer patients with 95 and 8,720 healthy males. Researchers took into account race, age as well as smoking, education or smoking cigarettes, body mass index consumption of calories from food, as well as the consumption of alcohol. They discovered that males who consumed the most boron had a lower chance of developing prostate cancer as than those who had the lower intake. They also noted the fact that a higher intake of boron in diet was linked to a lower chance of developing prostate cancer as a result of a dose-response relationship.

The findings did not just highlight the extraordinary, broad-spectrum of health benefits of consuming fruits, but found that boron specifically might be responsible for the protective effects.

Attracted by these findings that show a link between diet consumption of boron and a lower risks of prostate cancer scientists decided to investigate the possibility that boron supplements can help prevent prostate cancer. The initial animal research suggests that it is true.

In a tested animal model of prostate cancer observed that orally administering diverse amounts of a boran-based solution dramatically reduced the size of tumors. Also, it reduced levels of prostate-specific antibody or PSA--the main protein that is synthesized by the prostate gland. This suggests an explanation for the anticancer benefits.

The animal model used in this study the researchers administered different amounts of a boron-containing solutions to subjects in the test and discovered that the result was a decrease in prostate tumors' size between 25 and 38 percent. It was remarkable that PSA levels fell by a whopping 86 percentage to 89% for the boron-treated animals.

The results suggested that supplementation with boron might have both curative and therapeutic benefits, aiding to reduce prostate cancers and reduce concentrations of PSA.

Novel Protective Mechanisms

The discovery that additional boron can aid in shrinking prostate cancers and also reduce the levels of PSA7 are particularly thrilling. In the past, PSA was viewed primarily as a marker of blood for prostate cancer or infection or inflammation. But, new research suggests that PSA is a key factor in the development and metastasis of prostate cancer and thus, opening ways to prevent and treating this ailment by lowering PSA levels with nutrients like Boron.

Researchers now think that increased PSA causes the breakdown of proteins that surrounds prostate cell (called the extra-cellular matrix of protein) inside the prostate gland. This breakdown of cellular barriers caused by excessive PSA might be what allows prostate cancer to quickly invade healthy tissue and expand out beyond the prostate gland possibly resulting in death. These remarkable findings provide further insight into ways to stop or reduce the risk of developing prostate cancer by decreasing PSA levels.

The evidence published suggest that an increased intake of boron-containing substances may hinder PSA function and reduce the chance of developing prostate cancer through reducing intracellular calcium signals as well as storage.

Boron is becoming more well-known because of its ability to kill prostate cancer cells and reduce prostate-specific antigen or PSA. It also protects healthy cells from harm.

The levels of Boron in foods typically are very small.

A healthy intake of boron through supplements could help manage prostate cancer that could be fatal and help maintain optimal well-being.

Using Boron As Adjuvant Treatment

Numerous research studies have led scientists to believe that boron might be a specific therapy option to treat prostate cancer.

The less well-known PSA is the protein known as prostate-specific membrane antigen, or PSMA. Although PSMA is not confirmed as a reliable marker for prostate cancer, research studies have proven that PSMA is the main marker of PSMA in metastases and tumors in men suffering from prostate cancer is more prominent than PSMA for men who do not have prostate cancer.

In 2014, researchers published research on cells that focuses on the capacity of boron in reducing PSMA. They discovered that boron-rich substances showed significant levels of uptake from prostate cancer cells suggesting that boron-rich compounds could prove useful for the creation of a new category of treatment agents, such as boron neutron-capture therapy, or BCNT, to fight prostate cancer. BCNT is a form of injectable, non-invasive anticancer treatment that uses the element boron.

A further aspect of boron which is what makes it a particularly effective therapy agent is its capacity to inhibit development of prostate cancer cells, while permitting healthy prostate cells develop. The scientists know that these actions depend on the dose, but the mechanism that drives the targeted effects is in the process of being investigated.

An article published in 2014 was released in Tumour Biology but revealed that a substance that contained boron caused apoptosis which is the process of killing cells within prostate cancer cell. Researchers were able to discover that the boron-based agent affected the normal arrangement of prostate cancer cell's actin filaments that are thread-like protein fibers, which are an important part or building block for cells. The substance containing boron had additional cytotoxic effects or killed cells that included the decrease of telomerase activity within cancer cells. The researchers concluded that the boron contained in the chemical "could be an important agent for its therapeutic potential in the treatment of prostate cancer."

The more and more obvious conclusion is that making sure you have a daily intake of boron through supplementation -- and taking care not to rely on the small and wildly fluctuating amounts of boron present in food items from various farming regions -- is a crucial element of an approach to prevent prostate cancer as well as maintain healthy PSA levels.

Indeed, new research suggests that boron provides an additional level of protection against the symptoms associated with prostate cancer - in the bone.

The primary and most fatal risk of prostate cancer is it's ability to spread into the bone. This is the natural progression. Bone is the primary and primary site of 20% of all metastatic prostate cancer. Most often, they occur in the pelvis, spinal cord as well as the ribs, skull and the proximal femur.

The bone metastases cause bone remodeling, fractures, anemia and pain, which is a significant source of mortality and morbidity. Prostate cancer is classified by experts as "uniformly lethal once it has escaped the confines of the prostate gland." Tragically that is the case, the median lifespan for patients whose prostate cancer is spread to bone is about 40 months.

While more research is needed due to its incredibly targeted ability to stop the growth of cancerous prostate cells and protecting normal cells could be able to have a similar action against prostate cancerous cells that have spread into the bone. Through a greater boron-based supplementation program the cytotoxic effects -- when combined together with boron's ability to stop prostate cancer from developing from the beginning--could help to decrease the number of American mortality rate from the disease each year.

Boron can be described as a trace mineral which plays a vital role in the growth of plants and is incorporated into the diet of humans through eating of fruits and vegetables, particularly fruit, such as grapes, apples as well as avocados, veggies such as nuts, legumes and.

Although it is widely available in food items, taking sufficient amounts of boron from diet choices isn't easy. Why? The reason is that the quantity total of boron present in a single plant food is extremely low.

Apples, for instance, are believed as a great sources of boron. But, in order to reach the recommended minimum daily boron intake that is usually recommended for adults, it is recommended to consume around 2.4 pounds of apples per each day. That's more than 8 apples! It's not necessary to worry about exceeding the daily tolerable consumption (TDI) for Boron until you were able to consume 68 apples in the course of a single day!

Even more, in modern-day dietary practices, a lot of people can be deficient in boron due to just not eating sufficient amounts of fruits, vegetables and nuts. Even among people who consume a large amount of these food items the amount of boron they consume will greatly affect their local geology since the quantity of boron is largely depending on the amount of boron of the soil within the area where the food is grown. The local preference for particular products over others may lead to the human body having high or low levels of boron.

The importance of ensuring that you consume enough boron is ever more crucial as we get older. Since its inception, boron has been known for its vital contribution to ensuring the health of bones Scientists are becoming more excited over the growing evidence for its powerful ability to block the growth of prostate cancer.

9. CRUCIFEROUS VEGETABLES

Cruciferous veggies (broccoli, Brussels sprouts, collards, cabbage, cauliflower and mustard greens, kale (rutabagas, turnips, and watercress) contain four key chemotherapy-fighting compounds: Indole-3 carbinol (IC3), Diindolymethane (DIM), Phenethyl Isothiocyanate (PEITC) and the apigenin.

Indole-3-carbinol (I3C) is a compound with a variety of actions to help stop and reduce prostate cancer. It aids in activating detoxification pathways, stops cancer cells from growing, stimulates Apoptosis, regulates the expression of genes and shields DNA from harm, and regulates a range of signaling pathways in cells.

WebMD states:

Indole-3-carbinol has been used to reduce the risk of colon cancer, breast cancer and various types of cancer. It is believed that the National Institutes of Health (NIH) is studying indole-3-carbinol as a possible preventive drug and has begun to fund the clinical study of women's cancer prevention.

Indole-3-carbinol may also be prescribed for chronic fatigue syndrome, tumors in the vocal box (laryngeal papillomatosis) resulted from viruses, tumors within the respiratory tract (respiratory papillomatosis) due to viruses, unnatural development of cells within the Cervix (cervical dysplasia) as well as systemic lupus and erythematosus (SLE). Many people take indole-3-carbinol to stabilize the hormones "detoxify" the intestines and liver, as well as help strengthen the immune system.

Diindolymethane (DIM) has been shown to protect against prostate cancer by inhibiting the phosphorus-transferring enzyme Akt, inhibiting the master DNA-transcription regulator nuclear factor-kappaB (NF-kB)--and blocking the crosstalk between them. This is a new mechanism by that DIM hinders the growth of cells and triggers apoptosis within prostate cancer cells however, it does not affect non-tumorigenic prostate epithelial cell.

A study published in May 2013 PEITC was shown to inhibit the compound called

PROSTATE CANCER (P300/CBP-associated factor)--which also blocks androgen receptor-regulated transcriptional activities within prostate cancer cells.

When studying the human tumor cells researchers found that the extracts of vegetables apigenin reduces the growth of angiogenesis as well as cell growth. The effects were verified in an animal study that involved transplanting an androgen dependent line of prostate cancer cells from humans into mice bred as models for tumor development. A liquid suspension that contained either the apigenin drug or placebo was administered each day to the mice through a gastric tube for a period of eight to ten weeks. The administration of apigenin to mice - starting either two weeks prior to or after injection with the cells - inhibited the number of prostate cancer cells, in a dose-dependent fashion up to 59 percentage and 53% in both cases. Apoptosis-inducing in tumor xenografts was also observed. This study showed the exposure of prostate cancer cells to apigenin the culture for as short as 24 hours was found to slow the progression of cell cycles to a rate of 69%..

Researchers believe that these changes could be due to apigenin's influence on the IGF (insulin-like growth factors) Axis, which is responsible for functions of signaling in the proliferation of cells and death of cells. The research later revealed that apigenin inhibits the mobility and invasion of prostate cancer cells.

10. VITAMIN D

Recent years have seen many research studies have demonstrated that cancer-risk reductions are 50 percent or greater, in relation to the higher level of vitamin D. The people with higher levels of vitamin D are less likely to develop cancers of the prostate that are fatal, in addition to a reduced risk for other cancers. In 2011 Dr. Garland's group found that a vitamin D concentration that is 50 ng/ml has been related to a 50 percent less risk of developing breast cancer. (Similarly the study from 2007 released in American Journal of Prevention medicine9 found that a vitamin D concentration of over 33 ng/mL is associated with an increased risk of 50 percent of developing colorectal cancer.)

To attain a minimum safe amount of 40 ng/ml vitamin D, participants needed to consume between 1,000 IUs or up to 8000 IUs of vitamin D3 each day. This is far from the daily recommended allowance that is 600 IUs of vitamin D recommended for adults.

The dose that was added to ensure the 97.5 percent of the sample had a serum 25(OH)D minimum of 40 ng/mL was 9,600IU/day. It also found that a daily intake of as high as 40000 IUs daily is not likely to lead to toxic effects of vitamin D.

Numerous studies have shown that people who have higher levels of blood vitamin D lower the risk of developing cancer however, there was a gap that had not been addressed. was a double-blind placebo-controlled study which specifically examined the impact of high dose vitamin D supplementation (with calcium) on the incidence of cancer for people. It's the kind of research conventional medical professionals insist on doing in order to prove that the claims of a nutritional supplement (or medication) actually provides health benefits.

www.ingramcontent.com/pod-product-compliance
Lightning Source LLC
Chambersburg PA
CBHW051727020426
42333CB00014B/1196